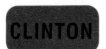

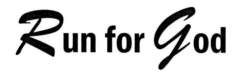

Run for God

THE 5K CHALLENGE

A practical guide to running and a 12-week training plan with a Christian focus.

Mitchell Hollis

CROSSBOOKS
PUBLISHING

CrossBooks™
A Division of LifeWay
1663 Liberty Drive
Bloomington, IN 47403
www.crossbooks.com
Phone: 1-866-879-0502

Scripture taken from the New King James Version. Copyright 1979, 1980, 1982 by Thomas Nelson, inc. Used by permission. All rights reserved. Scripture taken from the King James Version of the Holy Bible.

First published by CrossBooks 6/8/2010

ISBN: 978-1-6150-7253-8 (sc)
ISBN: 978-1-6150-7255-2 (hc)

Library of Congress Control Number: 2010908262

Printed in the United States of America
Bloomington, Indiana

This book is printed on acid-free paper.

If you require medical, fitness, or nutritional advice, you must contact your own health care professional. You should seek the advice of a doctor before starting any exercise routine.

This book may contain information relating to various medical conditions and their treatment, and an exercise/nutrition protocol. Such information is provided for informational purposes only and is not meant to be a substitute for the advice of a physician or health care professional. You should not use this information for diagnosing or treating a health problem or injury.

To make informed health care decisions, you should always consult your physician for your personal medical needs. Neither Run for God nor its agents, affiliates, partners, or licensors are providing these materials to you for the purpose of giving you medical advice.

For any questions about your health and well-being, please consult your physician.

Acknowledgments

I want to take a moment to thank God for all that He has done in my life, for being that still, small voice of reason in my head that has always pointed me in the right direction. At times I may not have listened, and at times I thought I knew better, but thankfully He is a patient God. His glory and peaceful nature will always shine through if only we allow it to.

Thank You, Lord, for all that You do!

Holly, Lane, and Landon, thank you for being the best family that any man could ask for. You have supported me 100 percent in everything that I have ever done and I can never repay you enough. I truly am the luckiest man on earth to have a family like you.

Holly, Lane, and Landon, I love you!

I want to thank my family, friends, and church family for all the kind words and encouragement you have given me. The first "Run for God" class was awesome, and I want to thank those of you who took a chance and committed to it. I am sure I got just as much or more out of that class as you did, and I want to thank everyone for sticking with it and finishing the race!

This would not have been possible without you!

Contents

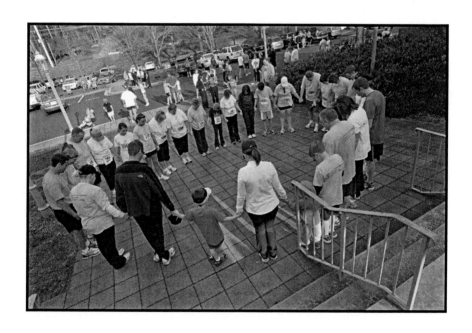

For additional books

or

small group packages (including teacher packages and merchandise)

visit

www.runforgod.com

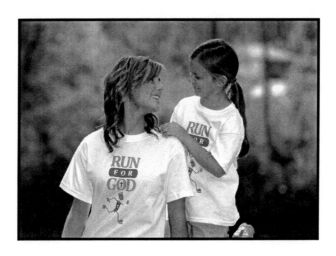

Week 1: Introduction

$\mathcal{W}$hy are you reading this book?

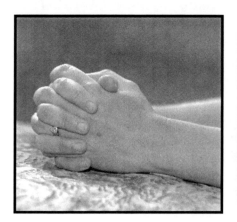 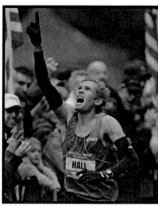

Before getting started, I would like you to think for a few minutes about this question. Write your answer below.

_____

_____

_____

_____

_____

_____

The answer that I have heard more than any is, "I need to get in shape." Although there is no right or wrong answer, it is a good idea to put your answer in writing so that you can refer to it from time to time, because it may change. You may have written "I need to get into shape," or, "I want to be around for my kids," or, "I want to grow closer to God." You may even have said all of the above.

Whatever your reason is, it is my hope and prayer that you will enjoy the sport of running and at the same time strengthen or even find your faith in the maker of all things, Jesus Christ.

*W*hy did I want to write a Christian running devotional?

You know, I don't know if I have fully gotten an answer to that question just yet. With that said, I do feel that I know what led me to where I am.

I started running in January 2007, and I was hooked from the moment I started. A few friends of mine were signing up for the Peachtree Road Race set for July 4, 2007, in Atlanta, Georgia. We all signed up and trained like a bunch of guys who thought we knew everything about the sport. We didn't have a plan, we didn't ask for advice, and we didn't think we needed any of that. We just knew that we had to cover 6.2 miles in the dead of summer and it didn't matter how we did it as long as we finished. Well, finish is about all we did. Most of the Kenyans (the fast guys) were already on a plane back to their home country by the time we crossed the finish line. Some of us were sore, some of us were so burned out we would never run again, and some of us had just caught a glimpse of something that we knew we could not get enough of.

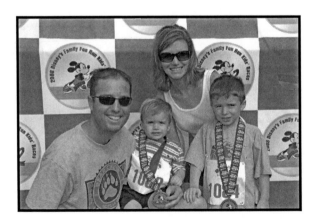

One of the guys who caught a glimpse was me. I came home complaining of hurting in places I had never hurt before and began trying to convince my wife Holly that we needed to do a marathon. At first she told me that I was off my rocker and that there was no way she could do a marathon. I finally convinced her that there was no way I could do a marathon right now either, but that in just six short months we could. The fact that we would do the Disney Marathon also helped a little.

So Disney it was. We signed up and started this adventure together, for better or worse. The next six months were tough. We would train together and separate. She would watch the kids while I ran, and then I would watch the kids while she ran. Whereas just a few months before, we would get a sitter so we could go enjoy dinner and a movie, we were now getting a sitter to go run. If it was a really special occasion, we would get a sitter, run the Chattanooga River Walk, go change and wipe off with a washrag in the local public restroom, and have some pizza downtown. Needless to say, we were committed!

It didn't seem like very long until it was time for Disney—Disney was here, ready or not. We felt good about our training and felt that we had done all we could do in such a short period of time. The only problem was that I had a stomach bug and really didn't know if I would even finish or not. With that said, almost six hours and what felt like ten restrooms later, we crossed the finish line. That night, every muscle in every part of our bodies hurt, but it was great! At least for me it was. Holly calls me a bit of a pain junkie. We felt like we had accomplished something, even if we did have to walk downstairs sideways to stop the sharp pains from shooting up our legs.

This experience only fueled my fire even more. I was already starting to think of what I could do next. I knew I had to improve my marathon time. What about ultra-marathons? And how about triathlons? Those looked fun, too. I was like a kid who had just learned that you really won't drown if you jump off the diving board. I wanted to do more a lot more.

In 2008 and 2009 I completed one 5K, five 10Ks, four 10 milers, three half marathons, two marathons, one 208-mile relay, one bike race, four triathlons, and one half Ironman. I got to where I loved endurance sports. It seemed like it was all I wanted to do or even talk about. Holly has supported me 100 percent and I cannot thank her enough for that. We even got our son Lane involved in Iron Kids, where he did great, even placing seventh at the national finals in Tucson, Arizona.

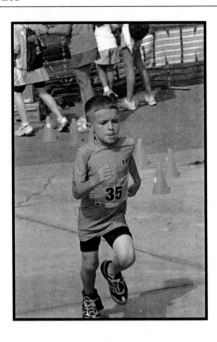

Through all that, I remained what I thought was faithful. I tried to be at church every time the doors were open, I often thought about how I could start a running ministry, I came up with the logo on the cover of this book almost two years before it was written, and I even had breakfast with my preacher from time to time. But I was often convicted of not spending enough time with God and in his word. I knew what God was saying, but I just didn't have enough time for him. I could spend fifteen to twenty hours a week in the final months before an Ironman event biking, running, swimming, and cramming my head full of secular music through my MP3 player, but I couldn't find fifteen to twenty minutes a week to be alone with God.

Well, I am convinced that God will do anything he wants to get your attention, even if it means getting your attention at times you least expect it. You see, in October 2009 I had just finished my first half Ironman and had just gotten back from Lane's Iron-Kids event in Tucson. Needless to say I had plenty to talk about. At our church's homecoming lunch I sat down beside some friends of mine, HR and Adrian Poe. I have known HR and Adrian for the better part of my life. They have always been solid, mature Christian leaders in my eyes, and they both also love to run. It seems like every time I get a chance to speak to them, that is where the conversation ends up, and this day was no different. HR and I were talking running, triathlons, Lane's race, and how I had committed to the Florida Ironman in 2010. After we had talked for a few minutes, HR looked at me, his face as serious and concerned as it could be, and said, "Mitch, don't let this become your God." Wow, I thought, where in the world did that come from? Here I am talking about running, traveling, and my kids, and HR is trying to give me pointers on my faith.

It wasn't until that night that HR's words really began to sink in. I started thinking back on the past few years at all the hints God had given me, like the idea of this running ministry, that I had just dismissed. God had put someone, *someone in my running world* in my path to get my attention and set me straight. Over the next few days I could not stop thinking about what HR had said and how he said it. Within a day or two I had dragged out the logo that I had sketched a few years ago. I knew I had to do one of two things: either stop using this sport that I love as an idol and an excuse, or use it to further God's kingdom.

You are not able to tell by reading this book, but I am not very comfortable sharing what God is doing in my life. This is where the logo comes in. A few weeks after that conversation with HR, I showed up on his doorstep one Saturday afternoon with some T-shirts that had this funny-looking stick man on them. They read, "Run for God."

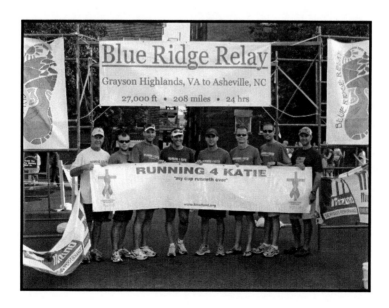

I remember when some friends of mine and I did the Blue Ridge Relay in 2008. We had team shirts made that said, "Running for Katie." Below that they said, "My cup runneth over." Katie was a young lady in our community who had died from acute myeloid leukemia. In the final months before her death she questioned why she was sick, she missed her daughter Merriwether during the months she spent in the hospital, she cried when the doctors told her the leukemia had returned, but she never rejected her faith in God's love for her. In her final letter to her friends and family, she implored them to tell someone about Jesus. I remember being amazed at how many people came up to us and asked about our shirts and the story behind them. I told HR and Adrian that story, and how it was the reason behind my stick-man shirts. I told them that from now on I would be sporting one of these shirts while running, whether on the treadmill at the local gym or in my next marathon. Maybe this would force me to get out of my comfort zone and share what God was doing in my life, because I knew people were going to ask about my funny-looking shirt.

As my pastor has said many times, I still felt that I needed to do more. I tried to figure out how I could get others to wear the shirts. Then I thought, *What better people to sport these fashionably correct shirts than people who love to run and love the Lord?* This also got me to thinking about the people over the years who have told me that they would like to get into running, but just didn't know where to start. That is where this book was born. I hope I can teach you a little about running and we can teach each other a lot about our enduring faith, all the while telling others about the great God we serve.

_____

_____

_____

_____

_____

_____

_____

_____

_____

_____

𝓜 ission Statement

**Preparing people to be better witnesses for Christ
physically, mentally, and spiritually**

Physically—Create a healthier you and make it possible to reach a new demographic of non-believers—potential believers!

> "Go ye therefore, and teach all nations, baptizing them in the name of the Father, and of the Son, and of the Holy Ghost:**20** Teaching them to observe all things whatsoever I have commanded you: and, lo, I am with you alway, *even* unto the end of the world."
>
> —Matthew 28:19–20 (KJV)

Mentally—Learn the discipline and endurance that it takes to "Run the Race Set Before Us"

> "Therefore we also, since we are surrounded by so great a cloud of witnesses, let us lay aside every weight, and the sin which so easily ensnares *us*, and let us run with endurance the race that is set before us."
>
> —Hebrews 12:1 (NKJV)

Spiritually—Learn always to give God the glory for all that we accomplish.

> "I will praise thee, O Lord my God, with all my heart: and I will glorify thy name for evermore."
>
> —Psalms 86:12 (KJV)

*O*bjectives

- To introduce the sport of running and to help you learn all that you need to know in order to make it enjoyable, satisfying, and rewarding.

- To understand the pitfalls that can come from letting anything become an idol to you.

- To understand the parallels of enduring a sport like running with enduring your faith.

- To understand how to become a better witness while doing something that you enjoy.

What are some things that typically become "idols"?

_____

What are some similarities between running and faith?

_____

_____

_____

_____

_____

_____

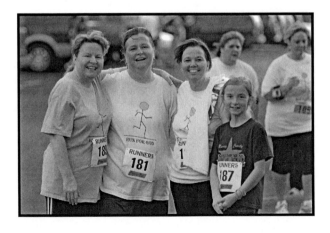

*D*isclosures

What qualifies me, "the author," to write this book?

I have never been asked this question before but I know that people have thought it. So I thought it would be better to answer this question right up front. The answer is nothing other than my God wanting me to do more. You see, there is nothing groundbreaking or earth-shattering about this book. I have simply taken what I feel the Lord has showed me and reduced it to writing. You can agree with me or you can disagree with me, but whatever you do, pray about it and agree with what God is telling your heart! Below I have outlined what I am and what I am not.

What I am	What I am not
Novice runner	Certified personal trainer
Young Christian	Bible scholar
Wanting to do more!	Physical therapist
	Nutritionist
	Medical doctor
	Preacher
	Psychologist

_____

_____

_____

_____

_____

_____

_____

_____

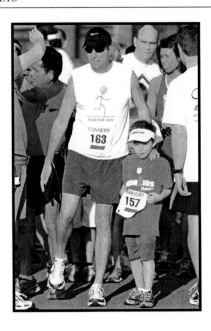

$\mathcal{R}$un for God Format

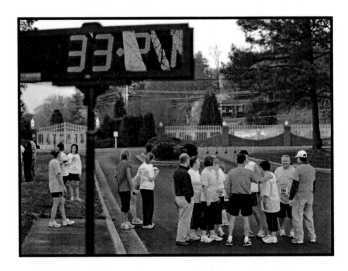

<u>Accountability Meetings</u>—Your group should hold meetings once a week. You can meet at your church, at a gym, or at someone's home, depending on

your group size. These meetings should consist of reviewing and discussing the weekly Bible study as well as new topics on running.

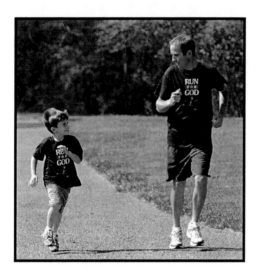

<u>Training Days</u>—Plan to train three days a week, preferably skipping a day between each workout: Tuesday, Thursday, Saturday or Monday, Wednesday, Saturday. It is a good idea to plan these workouts ahead just as if they were meetings or ball games. It is much easier to plan ahead than just "trying to fit it in." Also be sure to study your verses on the days you workout as well.

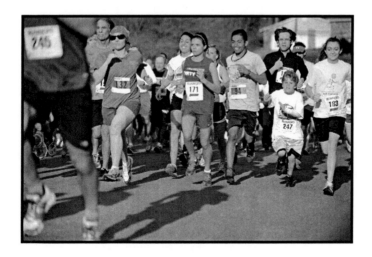

Race Day!—Count ahead twelve to fourteen weeks and book the date! Find a 5K that your group would like to attempt, and commit to it. Call the race director and discuss your plans. Ask if your group would be welcome, tents, screaming supporters, and all. I am sure the race organizers will support you 100 percent. Once booked, tell your friends, family, and church what you have done and why you have done it. Use this conversation to start your witness and your "Run for God" ministry.

_____

_____

_____

_____

_____

_____

_____

_____

_____

Some Topics We Will Cover

While we will not be able to cover everything there is to know about running, we will be able to hit the most important topics of the sport. Below are just a few of these topics.

Shoes	Injuries	Core Exercises
Stretching	Nutrition	Cross Training
Goals	Heart Rate	Pacing
Hitting the Wall	10 Percent Rule	Recovery
Hydration	Race Day Preparation	Sore vs. Hurting
Burnout	Runner's High	Types of Runs
Running Icons	Gear	Motivation

Running 101—Races?

All too often I find myself speaking to someone about this race or that race and they begin asking, "Now, how far is that?" Below are the most common race distances in the sport of running.

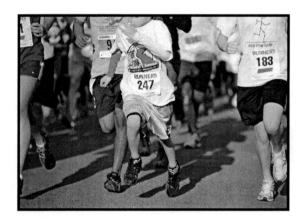

1 Mile Fun Run	1 mile
5K	3.1 miles (The most popular beginner race)
10K	6.2 miles
10 Miler	10 miles
Half Marathon	13.1 miles (The stepping stone to a marathon)
Marathon	26.2 miles (The goal of most serious runners)
Ultra-Marathon	Anything over 26.2 miles

$\mathcal{N}$eed to Know NOW!

Since you will begin your workouts this week, here are a few pointers to get you started on your journey.

1. **Set a Goal**—This is a must! Sign up for a race and commit. Tell your friends, family, and others what you have done and let them help hold you accountable.

2. **Start Slowly**—Do not try to do too much too fast. Listen to your body, follow your routine, and do not skip ahead! This only leads to burnout and possible injury.

3. **Shoes, Shoes, Shoes**—Make sure you have the correct shoe for your foot. Many beginner injuries can be avoided simply from getting the correct shoes for your foot. Find a reputable running store in your area that can perform a gate analysis, and seek their advice. We'll cover shoe selection in more detail in Week Three.

4. **Warm Up and Cool Down**—Warming your legs up gets the blood flowing where it needs to in order to avoid injury, and cooling down helps your body flush out toxins like lactic acid that prohibit speedy recovery.

5. **Rest, Rest, Rest**—Many people think that muscle is built while working out. In reality the opposite is true. Muscle fiber is torn and damaged during workout, while rest allows that tissue to repair itself and become more efficient. So, while you want to have quality workouts, you must have equal quality in you rest periods.

6. **Hydration is Key**—Keep your body hydrated, even when you are not exercising. Take a water bottle to work or school. Staying regularly hydrated will benefit you when it comes time to run.

7. **Think of Food as Fuel**—Now is not the time for a crash diet. While you may lose weight during this process, it is not the focus. We will address nutrition in more detail later on, but for now keep a good balance of carbs and protein in your diet and just eat sensibly!

8. **Get the Family Involved**—Nothing will make this journey easier than having the support of your family and friends. One way or another, get them involved!

_____

_____

_____

_____

_____

_____

_____

_____

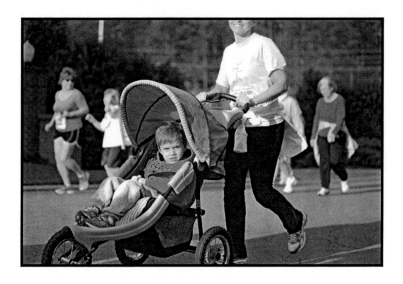

*W*here and When Should You Run?

Remember that a workout can fit into many aspects of your day, but the most important thing is to schedule it just like you do with everything else.

Where	**When**
In your neighborhood	Early, before the day starts
Secondary roads (always against traffic)	Lunch break
Parks	Afternoon, before dinner
Tracks (middle and high Schools)	While the kids are at ball practice
Sidewalks	On your way home from work
Treadmill	Make a day of it: take the kids and bikes

_____

_____

_____

_____

_____

_____

_____

*W*eek 1 Workout Plan

Workout 1—Start with a brisk 5-minute warm-up walk. Then al...nate 60 seconds of jogging and 90 seconds of walking for 20 minutes. Follow that with a 5-minute cool-down walk.

Total Workout = 30 Minutes

Workout 2—Start with a brisk 5-minute warm-up walk. Then alternate 60 seconds of jogging and 90 seconds of walking for 20 minutes. Follow that with a 5-minute cool-down walk.

Total Workout = 30 Minutes

Workout 3—Start with a brisk 5-minute warm-up walk. Then alternate 60 seconds of jogging and 90 seconds of walking for 20 minutes. Follow that with a 5-minute cool-down walk.

Total Workout = 30 Minutes

Remember to keep the following things in mind:

1. If you feel sore, keep going. If you feel pain, stop!

2. We are starting with jogging, not running. Keep a slow pace and let your body adjust to the new sensations over the next few weeks.

3. This may feel easy to some, but whatever you do, do not skip ahead. This is very tempting, but it can only lead to injuries and frustration.

*W*eek 1: Conclusion

First, I want to thank you for taking this journey with me. It is my hope and prayer that you will find the true joy that comes with this great sport that I love, a joy that can only be magnified if you do it to glorify our great and awesome God. Remember to keep your priorities in check and use others to help keep you accountable.

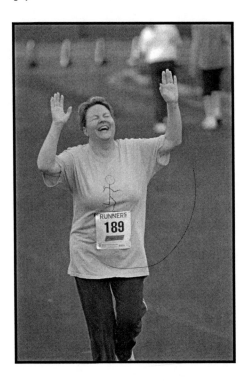

*T*ip of the Week

Accept the challenge.

"Everyone is an athlete. But some of us are training, and some of us are not."

—Dr. George Sheehan, runner/writer/philosopher

Week 2: Running the Race Before Us

𝒮tory

> "Therefore we also, since we are surrounded by so great a cloud of witnesses, let us lay aside every weight, and the sin which so easily ensnares *us*, and let us run with endurance the race that is set before us."
>
> —Hebrews 12:1 (NKJV)

Edwin Moses glided fluidly over the track of Oglethorpe University in Atlanta. He had no idea he was being watched by someone who had no idea who he was. The power of his stride captivated the dazzled observer. Though the spectator didn't know the runner, he was awed by what he saw.

The observer was playing tennis with a friend and asked, "Who is that?"

"That's the Olympic hurdler Edwin Moses," the friend said. "Allegedly he practices over here because Oglethorpe has the best track surface in the area."

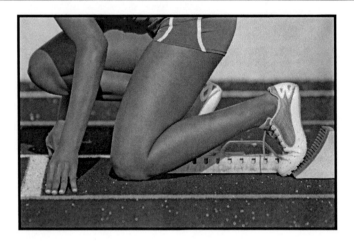

In his career, Edwin Moses won 107 consecutive finals and set the record for the 400-meter hurdles four times. Even though the observer had no idea who that runner was, he knew he was seeing someone special.

Surely, Christ was the same way. He was different from the typical person, and even those who didn't know him could tell he exuded something new. If Edwin Moses could manage to touch a naive life with the power and authority of his athleticism, surely Christ can touch our lives as well.

In a lot of ways, the experience of faith may be like a race. The athlete has to practice to compete. That practice may be grueling in nature at times. The athlete may experience boredom. He may have to deal with pain or injuries. In the spiritual race, the injury—the distraction—is sin. Temptation, doubt, fear, rebellion, and disinterest may sideline the believer. But it continues to be Christ who sets the pace and who calls us back onto the track. His life, death, and resurrection offer the victory over sin and death that wins the race.

The Holy Spirit is about the presence of God. People are touched by that presence. And in the race of life, which will eventually end, only One sets the pace of victory: Jesus Christ. We who are on the track stand in awe of what we see. It is he who enables us to run at all. The race of faith takes us to eternal life through God's wondrous hand.

Story by Douglas Bower

*D*iscussion

How can we be like a Christian Edwin Moses, one who teaches by his or her actions? _____

_____

_____

What kind of distractions do you often have to hurdle or stumble on in your Christian walk? _____

_____

_____

Who best helps you stay in the race for salvation? _____

_____

_____

_____

_____

_____

_____

_____

_____

*G*et in the Word

Workout 1—1 Corinthians 9:24

_____

_____

_____

_____

_____

Workout 2—2 Timothy 4:7

_____

_____

_____

_____

_____

Workout 3—Hebrews 12:1–3

_____

_____

_____

_____

_____

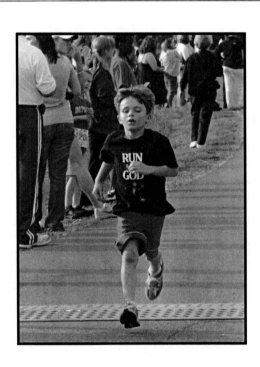

ear

Running Gear—The "Stuff" You Need

Running is an ideal sport for a lot of people because it does not involve investing in a great deal of expensive equipment or gear. With only a few basic pieces of gear, a novice runner can be ready to hit the streets. Compare this to other sports such as golf, rock climbing, or ice skating, which all involve the purchase of a great deal of expensive gear to even begin in the sport. You can also compare this to other team sports such as soccer, basketball, and football, which may not require a great deal of equipment but do require the participant to find and join an organized team or club. Any of these factors can make practicing the sport more time consuming, more expensive, and less convenient. However, running involves only minimal equipment and can be practiced by the individual either alone or in a group. Here we'll describe a few of the basic pieces of running gear required and a few pieces of more specialized gear which are not necessary but can make running more enjoyable or more effective.

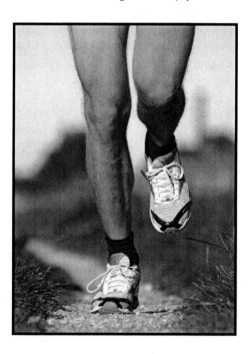

A good pair of sneakers is one of the most important pieces of gear for any runner. Quality sneakers are very important because they can help the runner to avoid injuries and can also keep him more comfortable while running. If you are unsure about what type of running shoe would be best for you, consider purchasing a running shoe from a store which specializes in selling sneakers to runners. The salespeople in these stores are likely to be much more knowledgeable than the personnel in a store where the sale of running shoes is not the main focus. Many of these specialized running stores even videotape customers running on a treadmill to evaluate their running style before making suggestions for possible sneaker selections. Once the salesperson has made these suggestions, they may ask the customer to run in each of these shoes to determine which shoe is best for the customer. The salesperson can make recommendations for which sneaker seems to be the best suited for the customer's style of running, but the customer will have to determine which sneaker feels the most comfortable.

Comfortable socks are also important to the runner. Socks that do not fit properly or are not designed specifically for running can cause the runner to develop blisters. If the socks do not fit properly, the fabric can rub against the foot while the person is running. Some popular types of socks designed specifically for runners have two layers. The inside layer fits closely to the foot while the outside layer fits more loosely. This design protects the foot because the inner layer acts as a buffer to any movement from the outer layer.

In addition to functional socks and shoes, a runner should also invest in quality clothing appropriate for the season. This should include shorts or pants and a long-sleeved or short-sleeved shirt of a thickness appropriate for the current weather conditions. Lightweight shirts with short sleeves are ideal for warm climates while heavier weight shirts with long sleeves are ideal for cooler climates.

Additionally, materials which help to wick moisture away from the skin can help to keep the runner cool and dry and can also help to prevent problems such as chafing, which may occur from moist clothing rubbing against the skin.

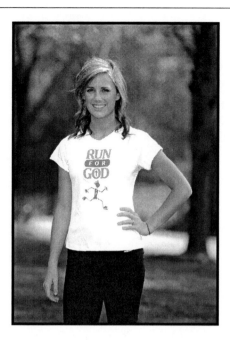

Other types of clothing can also be very useful for runners but are not exactly necessary to participate in the sport. This includes gear such as hats, rain gear, or clothing designed to resist the wind. These specific pieces of clothing can help a runner feel more comfortable in specific weather situations. For example, a hat with a wide brim can be very useful to runners who frequently run in very sunny weather. The hat can prevent sun from getting into the eyes and will protect the skin on the face from the damaging results of overexposure to the sun. Rain gear including waterproof pants and jackets can also be useful for runners who do not want to curtail their running just because it is raining. Effective rain gear will prevent the runner from becoming cold and wet while running in the rain.

Runners may also wish to invest in high-tech gadgets to aid them in their running program. Gadgets such as heart rate monitors, speed and distance monitors, and watches designed specifically for runners may not be necessary, but they can be very useful. A heart rate monitor is a device which typically includes a chest strap and a wrist unit. The chest strap transmits information to the wrist unit and the wrist unit displays useful information such as the heart rate, but may also include information such as the number of calories burned. Using a heart rate monitor can enable a runner to fine-tune his training program to ensure he is training at the right intensity. Speed and distance monitors allow the runner to track how far he has run and the pace at which he is running and also allow him to store this information for future use. The majority of these monitors utilize a GPS system to supply this information. Most of the high tech gadgets for runners can be rather expensive but many runners find these tools are very valuable during the training process.

By www.therunnersguide.com

---

*S*ome Typical Running Gear

Shoes	Gloves	Socks
Shorts	Shirts	Pain relief
Undergarments	MP3s	Nightwear
Water bottles	Hats	Mace
Magazines	Playlists	Ice baths
Watches	Heart rate monitors	Sunglasses

Questions?

_____

_____

_____

_____

_____

_____

_____

_____

_____

_____

_____

_____

_____

_____

_____

Week 2 Workout Plan

Workout 1—Start with a brisk 5-minute warm-up walk. Then alternate 90 seconds of jogging and 2 minutes of walking for 20 minutes. Follow that with a 5-minute cool-down walk.

Total Workout = 30 Minutes

Workout 2—Start with a brisk 5-minute warm-up walk. Then alternate 90 seconds of jogging and 2 minutes of walking for 20 minutes. Follow that with a 5-minute cool-down walk.

Total Workout = 30 Minutes

Workout 3—Start with a brisk 5-minute warm-up walk. Then alternate 90 seconds of jogging and 2 minutes of walking for 20 minutes. Follow that with a 5-minute cool-down walk.

Total Workout = 30 Minutes

Break it Down

Remember why you are doing this! It's okay to drown out your thoughts while running, but it is also a great time to have a conversation with the Lord. Next time you run, try turning off the MP3 and just talk—and especially listen—to God. You may be surprised at what you may hear.

Tip of the Week

Be a minuteman.

"The biggest mistake that new runners make is that they tend to think in mile increments—one mile, two miles, three miles. Beginning runners need to think in minutes, not miles."

—*Budd Coates, Olympic coach,*
four-time US Olympic Marathon Trials qualifier

Week 3: Run Your Race

Story

> "You ran well. Who hindered you from obeying the truth?"
>
> —Galatians 5:7 (NKJV)

On November 20, 2009 Gary Brasher attempted to accomplish something that most of us would never even consider, much less aspire to, when he completes a triple-iron triathlon. That's a full iron-distance triathlon every day for three consecutive days! He will swim, bike, and run his way over 422.6 miles in a 72-hour span! It is truly one of the most difficult sporting endeavors ever imagined.

I can still remember my first triathlon. It was many years ago now, and it wasn't anywhere near the iron distance. In fact, it was a "sprint" triathlon: .5-mile swim, 16-mile bike and 5K run. And as you can imagine, the name "sprint" indicates that you should basically be able to "go all-out" in a race of that distance. But for me, my first race was a debacle.

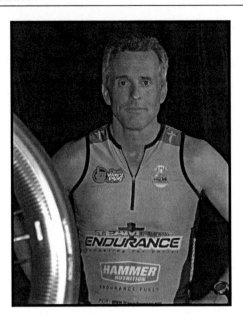

My goal was simply to finish. I had modestly trained for a few weeks and was pretty confident that I would be able to do it, but since it was all new to me, I really didn't know for sure. As I prepared for the race, I remember asking a number of friends that were experienced in the sport for advice. They were all a tremendous help, but alongside their training tips and technical advice came one important message from a friend who said, "Just run your race." In essence, "Don't worry about what everyone else is doing. Don't get sucked in to the pace of the rest of the racers. Simply run *your* race."

I was impressed with the simplicity of the advice, especially since many of these friends had completed in iron-distance events. They knew that I would be tempted to give in to the competitive spirit even though I was not physically prepared to go all-out. They also knew that my adrenaline would be high and that my mental approach to the event would have to control my emotional response to the electric race environment.

As the swim began, I foolishly threw their advice out the window and decided to try to stay stroke for stroke with the strongest swimmers. As a former competitive swimmer, I suddenly believed that I was sixteen again and could go out in front and avoid the congestion of all the bodies in the water. Needless to say, that was not the race strategy I'd planned! And the fact that the water was only sixty degrees gave me an instant shock experience that left me gasping for air—something that I wouldn't really recover from until I dragged myself from the water.

It didn't take long for me to have my first "near-drowning" experience as I completely ran out of gas. I nearly had to quit the race because I chose not to run *my* race. I got caught up in the excitement of the event and decided to abandon my plan and do what the other competitors were doing.

In Galatians 5:7, Paul asks the Galatians why they stopped running their race. Jesus had given them a specific race to run—one of freedom, grace, and love. Unfortunately, they got sucked back into following the requirements of the Law; they were burdened again by trying to earn God's favor. They'd lost the joy and peace that they'd received through the simple belief and trust in Jesus. Basically, they'd stopped running their race.

For me, it's so tempting to return to my old ways of trying to earn God's favor—to be performance-driven, to be "good enough," to follow the rules, to think that God is only pleased with me when I'm achieving or doing things just right. But this is a burden of slavery. And it's a lie. We are saved by grace, and we are changed by His Spirit. It's not something we do; it's something He alone can do in us.

So, don't get derailed by what someone else is doing. Don't let the emotion of the moment get you off course. Don't let your old ways of doing things make you abandon the new. Run *your* race. Stick to His plan and let God keep you on the path that leads to life.

Story by Jimmy Page, Fit4Ever, Sharing the Victory, FCA

𝒟iscussion

Do you ever find yourself looking for worldly answers rather than turning to the Bible? _____
_____
_____

Why do we seem to get on a "spiritual roll" sometimes and then fall flat at other times? _____
_____
_____

How can you better run "God's Race" rather than the world's? _____
_____
_____
_____

𝒢et in the Word

Workout 1—Acts 20:19–24

_____
_____
_____

Workout 2—Galatians 5:7

_____
_____
_____

Workout 3—Philippians 3:12–14

_____
_____
_____

*S*hoes

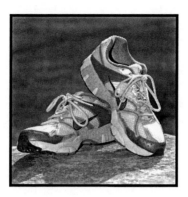

How to Choose Running Shoes

There are lots of running-shoe brands and styles on the market. While most running shoes feel comfortable when you're standing on the carpet in a sports store, the true test is after several miles on the trail or asphalt. You'll quickly realize that your perfect shoe has more to do with the shape of your foot and your running style than it does with the logo stitched on the side.

Road Runners or Trail Runners?

Road running shoes are designed for pavement and occasional forays onto packed surfaces with slight irregularities (fire roads, nature trails, wood-chip paths). Light and flexible, they're made to cushion or stabilize feet during repetitive strides on hard, even surfaces.

Trail running shoes are essentially beefed-up running shoes designed for off-road routes. They are enhanced with aggressive outsoles for solid traction and fortified to offer stability, support, and underfoot protection. If you routinely encounter roots, rocks, mud, critter holes, or other obstacles during runs, choose trail runners.

Tip: If you can't find a trail shoe with the right fit for your running mechanics, it's better to go with a road-running shoe.

Know Your Feet

Foot size: You probably know your shoe size already. But if you're unsure or if one foot is larger than the other, it's best to have your feet measured at REI or other shoe retailer with a Brannock device. (That's the flat metal tool with sliders that measure the length, width, and the toe-to-ball length of the foot.) Whenever possible, try the shoe on to see if it fits. Shoe lasts (which determines shoe sizes, described below) vary by manufacturer and even from one shoe model to another. You may need a half size or even a full size smaller or larger than you think.

Most men wear a D-width shoe while most women wear a B-width. You don't have to wear a gender-specific shoe—the lasts are basically the same. Men: Try a women's shoe if you have a narrow foot. Women: Try a men's shoe if you have a larger or wider foot. If the shoe fits, wear it!

Arch shape: Here's a simple way to find yours. As you get out of the tub, shower, or pool, take a look at the footprint you leave on the bathmat or cement. The shape of your footprint will indicate the type of arch you have. Your arch shape affects the way your foot moves as you run.

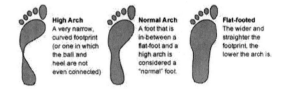

Biomechanics of Running

Your foot shape is closely related to its movement as you walk or run. The typical scenario: With every stride, your heel strikes the ground first. It rolls slightly inward and the arch flattens to cushion the impact. Your foot then rolls slightly to the outside and stiffens to create a springboard to propel your next step.

As runners, however, we each experience different levels of these sideways motions as we stride. The key characteristics:

Pronation is the foot's natural inward roll following a heel strike. Basic (neutral) pronation helps absorb impact, relieving pressure on knees and joints. It is a normal trait of neutral, biomechanically efficient runners.

Over-pronation is an exaggerated form of the foot's natural inward roll. It is a common trait that affects the majority of runners, leaving them at risk of knee pain and injury. Over-pronators need stability or motion control shoes.

Supination (also called under-pronation) is an outward rolling of the foot resulting in insufficient impact reduction at landing. Relatively few runners supinate, but those who do need shoes with plenty of cushioning and flexibility.

The illustration below shows these mechanics on a runner's left leg:

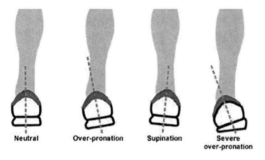

Neutral   Over-pronation   Supination   Severe over-pronation

How can you be sure which running style is yours? A podiatrist or physical therapist could undoubtedly tell you, but a simpler answer is probably in your closet. If you own a well-used pair of running shoes, check the wear pattern on the soles.

- If you have a neutral stride, shoe wear is centralized to the ball of the foot and a small portion of the heel.

- Over-pronation is identified by wear patterns along the inside edge of your shoe.

- Supination is marked by wear along the outer edge of your shoe.

Types of Running Shoes

Cushioning shoes provide elevated shock absorption and minimal medial (arch side) support. They're best for runners who are mild pronators or supinators. Cushioning shoes are also good for neutral runners during off-pavement runs. Reason: Minor irregularities in surfaces such as dirt roads give feet a little variety from the repetitive, same-spot strikes they typically experience on hard surfaces.

Stability shoes help decelerate basic pronation. They're good for neutral runners or those who exhibit mild to moderate over-pronation. They often include a "post" (see Shoe Construction 101, below) in the midsole. Due to their extra support features, virtually all trail-running shoes fall in the stability category.

Motion control shoes offer features such as stiffer heels or a design built on straighter lasts to counter over-pronation. They're best for runners who exhibit moderate to severe over-pronation.

Here are some general guidelines:

	Pronators	**Over-pronators**	**Supinators**
Foot mechanics	Normal inward roll	Excessive inward roll	Excessive outward roll
Foot shape	Low arch	Flat foot to low arch	Medium to high arch
Shock absorption in stride	Good	Good	Poor
Recommended shoe last	Semi-curved	Straight	Curved
Recommended type of shoe	Stability	Motion Control	Cushioning

*S*hoe Construction 101

Uppers

This refers to the upper part of the shoe above the sole.

- **Synthetic leather** is a supple, durable, abrasion-resistant material derived principally from nylon and polyester. It's lighter, quicker drying, and more breathable than real leather. Plus, it requires no (or very little) break-in time and therefore reduces the chance of blisters.

- **Nylon and nylon mesh** are durable synthetic materials most commonly used to reduce weight and boost breathability.

- **TPU (thermoplastic urethane) overlays** are positioned over the breathable shoe panels (such in the arch and the heel). These small, abrasion-resisting additions help enhance stability and durability.

- **Waterproof/breathable uppers** (e.g., Gore-Tex XCR or eVent) use a membrane bonded to the interior of the linings. This membrane blocks moisture from entering while still allowing feet to breathe. Shoes made with these membranes keep feet dry in wet environments with a slight trade-off in breathability.

Midsole Technology

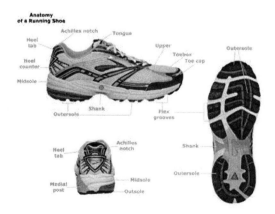

The midsole is the cushioning and stability layer between the upper and the outsole.

- **Synthetic leather** is a supple, durable, abrasion-resistant material derived principally from nylon and polyester. It's lighter, quicker drying and more breathable than real leather. Plus, it requires no (or very little) break-in time and therefore reduces the chance of blisters.

- **EVA** (ethylene vinyl acetate) is a type of foam commonly used for running-shoe midsoles. Cushioning shoes often use a single layer of EVA. Some will insert multiple densities of EVA to force a particular flex pattern.

- **Posts** are areas of firmer EVA (dual-density, quad-density, multi-density, compression-molded) added to create harder-to-compress sections in the midsole. Often found in stability shoes, posts are used to decelerate pronation or boost durability. Medial posts reinforce the arch side of each midsole, an area highly impacted by over-pronation.

- **Plates** are made of thin, somewhat flexible material (often nylon or TPU) that stiffens the forefoot of the shoe. Plates, often used in trail runners, protect the bottom of your foot when the shoe impacts rocks and roots.

- **Shanks** stiffen the midsole and protect the heel and arch. They boost a shoe's firmness when traveling on rocky terrain. Ultra light backpackers often wear lightweight trail runners with plates for protection and shanks for protection and support.

- **TPU** (thermoplastic urethane) is a flexible plastic used in some midsoles as stabilization devices.

Shoe Lasts

The "last" refers both to the shape of a shoe and also to the form, or mold, around which a shoe is constructed.

*W*hen referring to the shape of a shoe:

- A **straight last** is appropriate if you are an over-pronator or have a flexible, flat arch. It helps to control inward motion.

- A **curved last** is designed for under-pronators with rigid, high arches. The curved shape promotes inward motion.

- A **semi-curved last** represents the middle ground. It is appropriate for neutral pronators.

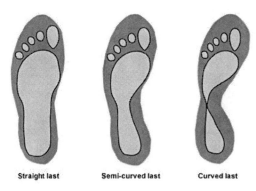

Straight last   Semi-curved last   Curved last

*W*hen referring to the shape of a shoe:

- **Board-lasted** shoes are made with a piece of stiff fiberboard glued to the upper and then to the midsole/outsole. These shoes offer the stability and motion control needed by over-pronators.

- **Slip-lasted** shoes are made by sewing the upper into a sock, which is then glued directly to the midsole/outsole without any board in between. These are flexible and well cushioned for the supinator.

- **Combination-lasted** shoes feature board-lasting in the rear half for motion control and support, which slip-lasting in front for cushioning and flex. This is the most common approach and can be used a wide range of foot types.

*O*ther Shoe Components

- **Heel counter:** This refers to the rigid structure around the heel. It provides motion control and is sometimes supplemented with a heel wedge, which adds support and cushioning to the heel. It can help those runners who are bothered by Achilles tendonitis.

- **Medial post or torsion bar:** These are located on the sides of shoes to help control excessive inward or outward motion. They are designed for the over-pronator or supinator.

- **Outsole:** The outsole is where the rubber meets the road, so to speak. Most road shoes are made with carbon rubber's hard, durable material in the heel. Blown rubber—which provides more cushioning—is often used in the forefoot. Trail runners tend to have all carbon rubber outsoles to better withstand trail wear, while road-racing shoes are frequently all blown rubber to reduce weight.

*F*it and Lacing Tips

When trying shoes on:

- **Try on shoes at the end of the day.** Your feet normally swell a bit during the day's activities and will be at their largest then. This helps you avoid buying shoes that are too small.

- If you **wear orthotics**, be sure to bring them along. They impact the fit of a shoe.

- Consider **custom footbeds (insoles)** such as Superfeet. Shoe manufacturers tend to provide generic insoles with their shoes since many runners use orthotics or, increasingly, custom footbeds. By using a custom footbed, you get improved cushion, stability and a better fit. These are great for people with back problems or who run long distances.

Lacing techniques for various foot types:

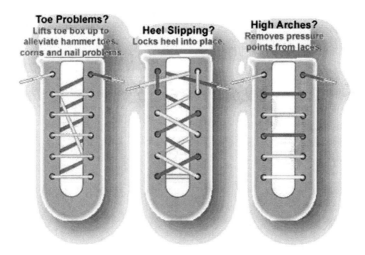

Shoe FAQs

Q: How snugly should a running shoe fit?

A: You should have a thumbnail's length of extra space in the toebox. This helps you avoid losing toenails since your toes won't jam against the end when running downhill or when your feet swell. The width should be snug but allow a bit of room for your foot to move without rubbing. Laces should be snug but not tight.

Q: What is the typical lifespan of a running shoe?

A: In general, a pair of running shoes should last between 300 to 500 miles of running (three or four months for regular runners). This varies depending on your running mechanics. Take a look at your shoes. While the uppers will often look good, check the midsole and outsoles to see if they are compressed or worn.

Q: If I wear an orthotic to correct my pronation, do I still need a motion-control shoe?

A: You may be okay with a neutral shoe, but a motion-control shoe offers the most additional support.

Q: Can I use a road shoe for running trails?

A: Absolutely, just keep in mind that a trail shoe will give you more traction on rough or loose surfaces than a road shoe.

Q: If I supinate, can I wear a shoe that is for over-pronators?

A: You shouldn't. It's best to go with the shoe that coordinates with your body mechanics to avoid any injuries.

Q: Is it okay to do a race or long run while wearing new shoes?

A: The best approach is to do a short run first to see how your new shoes feel. You want to make sure the shoe is right for you before hitting a trail or pounding the pavement in a race.

By Linda Ellingsen
Article reprinted with permission of REI.

Questions?

_____

_____

_____

_____

_____

_____

_____

_____

_____

*W*eek 3 Workout Plan

Workout 1—Start with a brisk 5-minute warm-up walk. Then alternate 90 seconds of jogging and 2 minutes of walking for 20 minutes. Follow that with a 5-minute cool-down walk.

Total Workout = 30 Minutes

Workout 2—Start with a brisk 5-minute warm-up walk. Then alternate 90 seconds of jogging and 2 minutes of walking for 20 minutes. Follow that with a 5-minute cool-down walk.

Total Workout = 30 Minutes

Workout 3—Start with a brisk 5-minute warm-up walk. Then alternate 90 seconds of jogging and 2 minutes of walking for 20 minutes. Follow that with a 5-minute cool-down walk.

Total Workout = 30 Minutes

*B*reak it Down

Remember, to be a runner you must have the right equipment, be determined, faithful, diligent, and focused. Same goes for being a Christian!

*T*ip of the Week

Wear good running shoes.

"Don't skimp on your shoes. A good pair of running shoes should last you 400 to 500 miles and is one of the most critical purchases you will make."

—*John Hanc, author*
The Essential Runner

Week 4: Free to Run

*S*tory

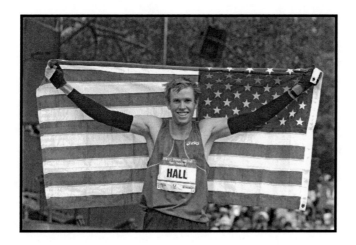

Tucked neatly between peaks of California's San Bernardino Mountains is the quiet reservoir town of Big Bear Lake, population 5,500. It is a cozy ski resort town full of log-cabin charm, the kind of place that begs visitors to forget that the turbulence of Hollywood sits at its feet only 100 miles away.

It was in this quiet town that an Olympic quest began. US marathon runner Ryan Hall was only fourteen years old when he stared out at the lake through his parents' car window and was filled with a vision—a vision to run. His school had no cross country team at the time, but he'd seen his dad do it before. He wanted to run the fifteen miles around the lake. But it wasn't as much a personal challenge as it was a calling—a prompting of the Holy Spirit. *"Do this, Ryan,"* He seemed to say. *"Do this for Me."*

So Hall ran. He ran down Big Bear Boulevard, across the bridge, up the north shore trail through Fawnskin, over the dam on the west side and back home. And the course of his life forever changed.

What had been a typical adolescence of basketball, school, and popularity gave way to a life of endurance, discipline, and faith: faith that he could always go one more mile; faith that he could always go a second faster; faith that his Father would run with him every step of the way.

Now a decade after that first run around the lake, Hall has emerged as one of the most gifted endurance athletes the United States has ever produced. After a notable cross country career at Stanford University, Hall distanced himself from the elite running pack when he broke the American half marathon record in 2005 with a time of 59:43. Then, in just his first attempt at a full marathon, Hall stunned the running world by turning in the fastest debut marathon time ever by an American athlete (2:08:24) at the 2007 Flora London Marathon—an event that he repeated [in] April only to beat his previous time by more than two minutes.

But it was his second marathon that truly captured the attention of his country and endeared him as the future of US distance racing. On November 3, 2007, Hall took to the streets of New York City for the Olympic Trials and not only won the race by more than two full minutes, but also broke the US Olympic Trials record. With arms lifted in praise to God, he blazed across the finish line and into an eleven-year-old dream of representing his God and his country in the Olympic Games.

*****

The Bible makes an incredible number of references to the sport of running, paralleling it to the lives of believers and the journeys of exhaustion, pain, and dedication all Christ-followers must experience.

Ryan Hall has a favorite: Isaiah 40:31. *"... but those who trust in the Lord will renew their strength; they will soar on wings like eagles; they will run and not grow weary; they will walk and not faint."*

"That embodies how I feel out there running," Hall said, as he reclined in his deck chair on a chilly 40-degree day in Big Bear earlier this year. "I feel like it's the Lord running through me, and I feel like I'm under His wings—like He's the One doing the work and I'm just catching a ride."

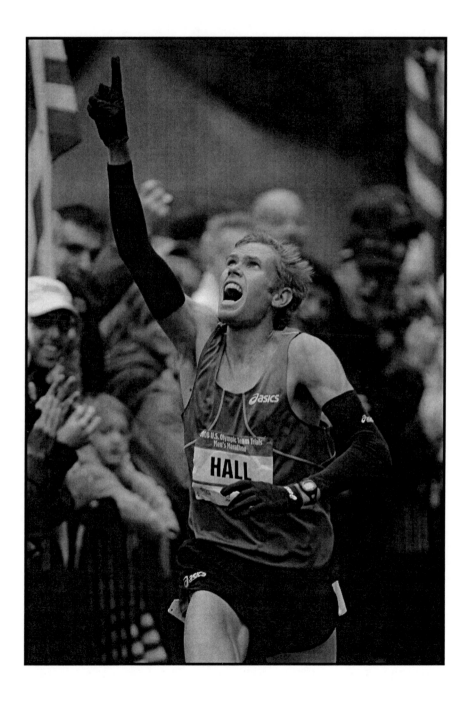

The mature attitude Hall carries about running is one that has been earned through trial and error. It hasn't always been an easy downhill run with the wind at his back. Quite the opposite. If anything, Hall has endured many miles of his journey going uphill against the wind.

After earning title after title in high school and entering college with great expectations, Hall became single-minded in his pursuit of running goals, specifically qualifying for the Olympic Games. He started a physical countdown to the 2004 Olympics 1,100 days in advance and made it his sole purpose and passion to run in Athens.

_____

_____

_____

_____

_____

_____

_____

_____

_____

_____

"I could sum it up in one word," he said. "Obsession."

But trying to handle the emotional and physical demands of his goal and still keep up with faith activities, academics, and a social life was more than he could handle. It wasn't long before his mind and body began to rebel.

Hall recalls with stark clarity being so burned out that he could barely crawl out of bed. There were mornings when he'd wake up, try desperately to go for a run only to get 800 yards, give up, and walk back home.

"There wasn't anything wrong with my body; it was just emotionally and spiritually I was wrecked," he said. "The Olympics had been a dream that I'd had for a really long time, and this was my first real crack at it. I was at the age where I expected to be in the Olympics, and I was really optimistic about my chances. But that's when my world just came tumbling down."

Instead of competing in the 2004 Games, Hall—by that time, tired, frustrated, and out of shape—wound up watching the Olympic Trials with his little brother from their parents' van while camping along the Sacramento River—not the experience he had hoped for or expected.

But as the phrase goes, in man's limitation lies God's occasion. The plan had not changed. God's calling on Hall's life was still to run, but there were invaluable lessons that stood between where he was and where God needed him to be.

*****

_____
_____
_____
_____
_____
_____
_____
_____
_____
_____
_____
_____
_____
_____
_____
_____
_____

Step one of Hall's journey was to remove running as an idol in his life. Instead of living, sleeping, eating, and breathing to be the best runner in the world, he had to learn to live, sleep, eat, and breathe for Christ above all. Having accepted Christ as a young man and being the product of a Christian home, Hall's running had always been intertwined with his faith, but not to the point where it was a genuine offshoot of his devotion to the Lord.

At the end of a fraying rope, Hall removed himself from Stanford University for a semester to ponder his future.

"I needed to figure out where God was calling me to be and what God was calling me to do," Hall said. "I wasn't sure it was running anymore."

His burnout continued back home in Big Bear, but slowly, things began to change. Away from distractions, Hall was better able to hear the voice of God, and soon, it all made sense.

What Hall realized was that it had never been about him or the goals he'd set—they never should have been the point. The Lord had given him the gift of endurance and had a plan to use that gift, but for His purpose. The only responsibility that remained on Hall's shoulders was to run in such a way as to maximize that gift. In return, God would supply the results.

That decision also meant that Hall was free from the intense pressure to achieve anything. He simply had to run for Christ.

"I finally surrendered it all and said, 'Whatever You want to do with it, do it. If You want to take me to the Olympics, great. If You don't, that's great, too,'" he said. "There was something very freeing about giving my gift back to God. I believe He's given us all special gifts, but I don't think we can develop them and enjoy them how we're intended to until we give them back to Him."

In almost every marathon, there is an invisible wall. Hall had just broken through his.

Hebrews 12:1, which paints a liberating picture of a runner casting off everything hindering his forward progress, suddenly came to life as Hall emerged from the bonds of pressure and began to run with freedom and joy.

Finally, he was back on track.

"Being free to run means not carrying the burdens of this world," Hall said. "It's the freedom to not have to achieve something—to be able to just go out and do it for the love of doing it. To do it because I feel like God's created me to do it. To do it as my act of worship to God."

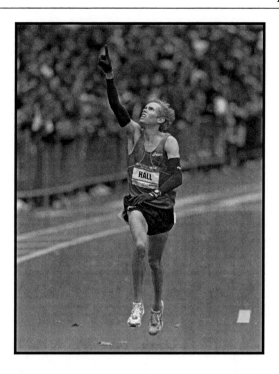

New York City, November 3, 2007. It's early in the morning. Most of the city is still sleeping off its Friday night, but there is commotion in Central Park. Thousands of spectators line the running path as a select group of the fastest distance runners in the country glide swiftly around the five-mile loop.

The race has only been underway a short time, and the pack remains close together. It is doubtful that anyone hears the song of praise emerging from two of the lead runners.

Hall and fellow believer/elite runner Josh Cox are striding along together, in step with each other and in step with God.

"Savior, He can move the mountains. My God is mighty to save; He is mighty to save."*

They sing as best they can, exhaling a chorus of praise. It is a special time for these two men. They are doing what their Lord has created them to do in that moment: worshipping Him body, mind, and spirit.

For Hall, it was a day he'd dreamed of for years, but it was nothing like he'd imagined. The victory he'd sought so passionately years ago seemed a minor footnote. He had a different purpose now.

"I honestly didn't have the goal to win the Olympic Trials," he said, throwing caution to every running stereotype. "My goal was to praise God. And that was very important because I still struggle with getting too into running and too obsessed with what I'm doing. I have to hold myself back from that, and the way I do that is to just have one single goal: to praise God with every single step and with every single race."

*R*yan Hall Q&A

All those miles on the open road left only to his thoughts have paid off for Ryan Hall. The guy is sharp! Check out some of the Q&A from Sharing the Victory's *interviews:*

STV: In the Bible there are so many verses about running, and it is used many times as a metaphor for our spiritual lives. Why do you think running is such a great spiritual parallel?

RH: I think it's because it's a challenge. Especially in America, we want to be comfortable and we want to have things come easily to us, and running's not like that. When you're out there training, you're pushing yourself through pain. That's the whole deal with running: How hard can you push yourself and how hard can you train? I think that's a lot like our spiritual walk. You have to continue to challenge yourself, and you can't expect it to come easily.

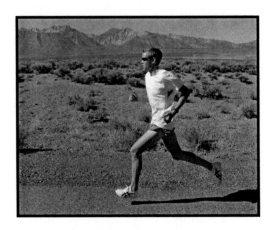

And while there are times that are hard, there are also times that are just fun. Like for me, the Olympic Trials race was just fun. That was one of the most amazing races I've run; I felt awesome the whole time and enjoyed the entire race. It was one of the best two-hour time periods of my life. And I think it's like that with our spiritual walks, too. We're going to go through the valleys—the high times and the low times—but we just have to keep putting one foot in front of the other.

STV: FCA's Camp theme this year is "Get Focused," and it's based on Philippians 3:12–21, which talks about forgetting what is behind and pressing on for Christ. What significance does that concept have in your life?

RH: That's huge. I've come back to that over and over again—the concept of forgetting what's behind. It's a difficult one to master. Like, even this year, I didn't have the race that I wanted to have at the Cross Country Championships. It's easy to let things like bad races discourage us and make us give up, but if you're able to forget and move on, you won't give up on what God's called you to do.

God's given us all a task to do here on earth, and in accomplishing that task we need to put our failures behind us and continue to move forward. A lot of being a great athlete is just getting back up. I've always wondered what it was like to be an Olympian. What's an Olympian like? What makes them tick? And now, [I realize] I'm a normal person just like everyone else. I've just gotten my butt kicked a bunch of times and gotten back up every single time. And that is a big part of running and a big part of life. It's just getting back up.

One of my favorite verses in the Bible is Proverbs 24:16 (NIV), which says, "… a righteous man falls seven times, he rises again …" I love that verse, and I think about it all the time because I fall all the time. Whether it's spiritually or physically or whatnot, I'm always challenging myself to get back up and move forward.

*By Jill Ewert, **Sharing the Victory,** a publication of FCA*

_____
_____
_____
_____
_____
_____
_____
_____
_____
_____
_____
_____
_____
_____

*D*iscussion

Why do you think that we as Christians often hit a "spiritual wall?"

_____
_____
_____
_____

How do we overcome that wall? _____

_____
_____
_____

What does getting past that spiritual wall feel like? _____

_____
_____
_____
_____
_____
_____
_____
_____

_____

_____

_____

_____

_____

_____

_____

_____

_____

*G*et in the Word

Workout 1— Proverbs 24:16

_____

_____

_____

Workout 2— Isaiah 40:31

_____

_____

_____

Workout 3—Psalms 119:32

_____

_____

_____

$\mathcal{S}$tretching/Core Exercises

Repeat each stretch one to three times:

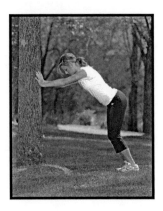

1. Wall Pushup 1

Stand about three feet from a wall, feet at shoulder width and flat on the ground. Put your hands on the wall with your arms straight for support. Lean your hips forward and bend your knees slightly to **stretch your calves**.

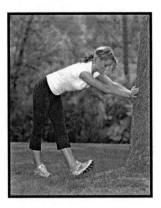

2. Wall Pushup 2

From the previous position, bend forward to lower your body to waist height. Bring one foot forward with your knee slightly bent. Lift the toes of the front foot to **stretch the muscle under the calf**. Stretch both legs.

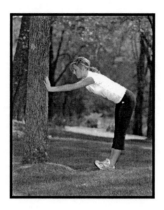

3. Wall Pushup 3

Put your feet together, rocking back on your heels with your hands on the wall and your arms straight to form a jackknife with your body. **This stretches your hips, shoulders, and lower back.**

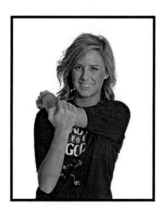

4. Back Scratch

Grab your elbow with the opposite hand and gently push the elbow up and across your body until your hand reaches down to "scratch" your back. Gently push on your elbow to guide your hand down your back as far as it will comfortably go, stretching your triceps and shoulders. Stretch both arms.

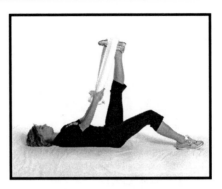

5. Hamstring Stretch

Lie down with one leg straight up in the air, the other bent with foot flat on the ground. Loop a towel over the arch of the lifted foot, and gently pull on the towel as you push against it with your foot. Push only to the point where your muscles contract. Stretch both legs.

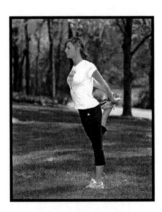

6. Heel to Buttock

Stand on one foot, with one hand on a wall for balance. Hold the other foot with the opposite hand and raise the heel of the lifted foot to the buttocks (or as close as comfortably possible), **stretching your quadriceps**. Keep your body upright throughout. Change legs and repeat.

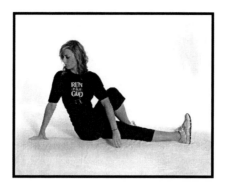

7. Hip and Lower Back Stretch

Sit on the ground with your legs crossed. Lift your right leg and cross it over the left, which should remain bent. Hug the right leg to your chest and twist the trunk of your body to look over your right shoulder. Change legs and repeat (i.e. looking over your left shoulder).

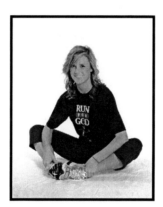

8. Groin Stretch

Seated, put the soles of your feet together. With your elbows on the inside of your knees, gradually lean forward and gently press your knees toward the ground.

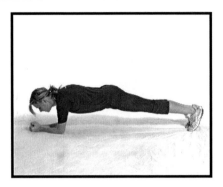

9. Planks

The plank exercise is a great way to build endurance in the abs and back, as well as in the stabilizer muscles. To do it right:

1. Lie face down while resting on the forearms, palms flat on the floor.

2. Push off the floor, raising up onto toes and resting on the elbows.

3. Keep your back flat, in a straight line from head to heels.

4. Tilt your pelvis and contract your abs to prevent your rear end from sticking up in the air.

5. Hold for 2 to 90 seconds, lower, and repeat for 1–3 reps.

Questions?

_____

_____

_____

_____

_____

_____

_____

_____

_____

Week 4 Workout Plan

Workout 1, 2 and 3

Brisk 5-minute warm-up walk

Jog 90 seconds

Walk 90 seconds

Jog 3 minutes

Walk 3 minutes

Jog 90 seconds

Walk 90 seconds

Jog 3 minutes

Walk 3 minutes

5-minute cool-down walk

Total Workout = 28 Minutes

Week 4 Conclusion

Remember that we often get so busy in doing what we think God wants that we miss Him totally. We pray, pray, pray, but sometimes we need to slow down or even stop, and just LISTEN!

Tip of the Week

Take the "talk test."

The "talk test" means running at a pace comfortable enough that you can carry on a conversation with a training partner; but not so easy that you could hit the high notes in your favorite gospel song.

Week 5: The Hay is in the Barn

Story

> "My son, if you receive my words, and treasure my commands within you ... Then you will understand the fear of the LORD, and find the knowledge of God."
>
> —Proverbs 2:1, 5 (NKJV)

The day before last year's Kansas City marathon, I was meeting with Chris Anderson, our national director of FCA's Endurance Ministry. I was fired up for the race but a bit anxious about trying to run a personal record. As I was reflecting back on my training leading up to the race, I mentioned to him that I wished I'd done more long runs, more speed work, more conditioning, more everything. I was feeling the pressure. He smiled real big, leaned across the table and said, "Dan, at this point, the hay is in the barn. The race is tomorrow. Nothing you can do now." Focused on the race and not fully understanding his point, I thought to myself, "I don't have hay or a barn." He helped me out and explained that it meant the work had been already done and that there was no more time to cram. The formal training was over and there was no looking back—nothing more to do but execute on race day. Now I just had to use what was stored up and let it work itself out during the race.

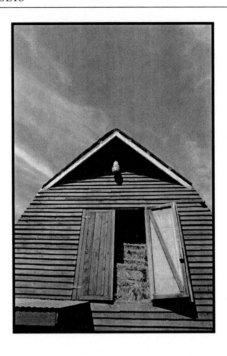

As I raced the next day, I thought about using my hay and the investment I'd made over the months leading up to the race. The hours of training that I had put in now revealed whether or not I would PR. Those days I didn't feel like getting in the 20-mile training runs but did anyway were paying big dividends. As I cranked away in the last two miles of the race, I began to pull away from the group that I had been running with the entire race. I immediately thought back to the race the year before when my pack had left me in the dust as a result of my lackluster training. There had been no hay in the barn when I'd needed it. But this year was different. There was plenty of hay in the barn, and I was blessed with a PR. It was good day of running! I ran well on race day because I trained well months before.

Ever since that day, Chris' comment has often rattled around in my head. It's a powerful principle. I thought if this is true for my running life, it is even truer for my spiritual life. The spiritual hay is the Word of God, and the barn is my heart. Sometimes, however, we fall into the trap of wanting a spiritual PR without putting in the spiritual investment. I know for me that I sometimes want God to show up and do something miraculous without me having to invest the time to know him better. We think God will do His miraculous thing anyway, so what does it matter if I really press in and get serious about my walk? If I love Jesus more, does that change anything? And what does it even look like to love God more? If I connect with Him daily and rely on Him to direct me throughout the day, will it really make a difference?

> Proverbs 2:1 says to store up His commands. (i.e. Put hay in the barn!) We must dive into the Word so that our lives can be governed by truth and motivated by love. For me, spending daily time in the

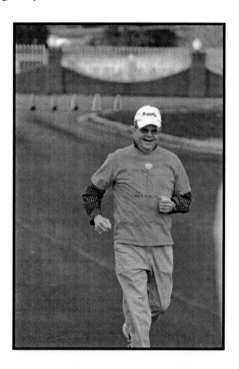

Word is more about the future than today. Yes, I draw on His Word daily, but when it comes to my training times, it always comes back to what I invested months earlier. I have come to realize that I will never regret spending too much time with Jesus. You never hear people saying they invested too much time in their walk with the Lord. Instead, I hear almost daily from followers of Christ, "I wish I could spend more time in the Word, but …" We all have our reasons, but not one of them is a good one.

Today, ask yourself if there is spiritual hay in your heart. Have you put in the time? Are you expecting great things with no spiritual sweat? Would you make varsity without ever picking up the ball? At mile 24, what would you have left in the tank? Start today. Carve out the time. Make an investment. Go deeper. It might be the single most important decision you make! When the strain comes, will you be able to draw on God's commands that were stored up months ago? Start putting spiritual hay in the barn today. Your tomorrow depends on it.

Story by Dan Britton, FCA

_____
_____
_____
_____
_____
_____
_____
_____
_____
_____
_____

*D*iscussion

How do you put spiritual hay in your barn? _____
_____
_____
_____
_____

What are your excuses for not spending more time in God's Word? _____
_____
_____
_____
_____

How do you make sure you don't fall into a rut when you spend daily time with the Lord? _____

_____

_____

_____

Why does your tomorrow depend on today? _____

_____

_____

_____

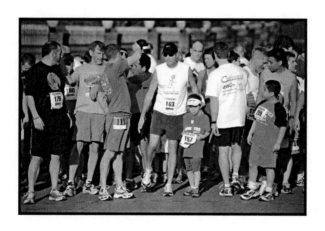

𝒢et In the Word

Workout 1—Deuteronomy 5:29

_____

_____

_____

Workout 2—John 14:21

_____

_____

_____

Workout 3—Hebrews 6:1

_____

_____

_____

Extra Credit—1 John 3:22

_____

_____

_____

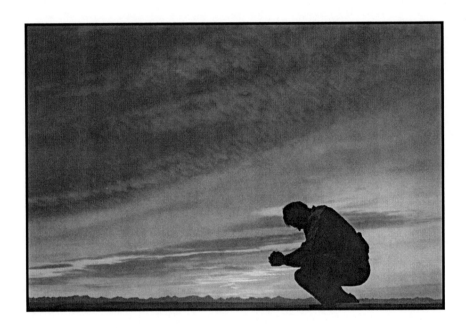

*I*njuries / Injury Prevention

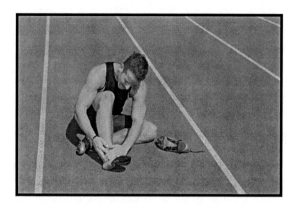

Once you've been running for a while, you may eventually have to deal with the pain and inconvenience of an injury. Most common running injuries are due to overuse, overtraining, improper shoes, or a biomechanical flaw in body structure and motion. The good news is that you can prevent many running injuries. Follow these steps to keep yourself on the road.

Avoid the "terrible toos." Many running injuries are a result of overtraining: too much intensity, too many miles, too soon. It's important to go easy when adding mileage or intensity to your training. You shouldn't increase your weekly mileage by more than 10 percent each week. You can still push your limits, but you'll have to take a gradual and patient approach. By building up slowly, you can save yourself pain and frustration, and still reach your goals. Let common sense and a smart training schedule determine how much you should be running.

Treat your feet right. Be sure that your shoes aren't worn out and that you have the right model for your feet and running style. The wrong shoe can actually aggravate existing problems, causing pain in your feet, legs, knees or hips. Wearing shoes that have lost their cushioning may also lead to injury. Go to a specialty running shop that can properly fit you for running shoes, and replace them every 350 to 500 miles. If you have a biomechanical problem with your feet, you may also look into getting fitted for heel lifts or orthotics.

Find the right surface. Once you have the right shoes, you want to make sure you're using them on the best surface. Ideally, you want the ground to absorb shock, rather than passing it along to your legs. Avoid concrete as much as possible: It's about ten times as hard as asphalt, and is a terrible surface for running. Try to find grass or dirt trails to run on, especially for your higher mileage runs. Consistency is important, too, because a sudden change to a new running surface can cause injuries. You'll also want to avoid tight turns, so look for slow curves and straight paths.

Stay loose. A regular stretching program can go a long way toward injury prevention. Be diligent about stretching after your runs—your body will make you pay if you get lazy about it.

Keep your balance. Injuries sometimes pop up when you're paying too much attention to your running muscles and forgetting about the others. For example, knee injuries sometimes occur because running strengthens the back of your legs more than the front of your legs. Your relatively weak quads aren't strong enough to keep your kneecap moving in its proper groove, which causes pain. However, once you strengthen your quads, the pain will often go away.

Make sure you're ready to return. To prevent re-injury, ease back into training with water running, cycling, or using an elliptical trainer. Overtraining is the number one cause of injuries, so try to remember that progress takes time.

Question: How can I avoid and treat muscle cramps?

I'm training for a marathon and towards the end of my long runs, my legs muscles start to cramp up. How can I prevent muscle cramps?

Answer: Muscle cramps are often the result of dehydration, so it's important that you make sure you're hydrating properly before, during, and after your runs.

Before Runs: An hour before you start your run, try to drink 16 to 24 ounces of water or other non-caffeinated fluid. Stop drinking at that point, so that you can void extra fluids and prevent having to stop to go to the bathroom during your run. To make sure you're hydrated before you start running, you can drink another 4 to 8 ounces right before you start.

During Runs: The general rule of thumb for fluid consumption during your runs: Take in 6 to 8 ounces of fluid every 20 minutes during your runs.

During longer runs (90 minutes or more), some of your fluid intake should include a sports drink (like Gatorade) to replace sodium and other minerals (electrolytes) lost through sweat. Muscle cramping often occurs because of electrolyte imbalance, so it's critical that you replace your electrolytes.

After Runs: Don't forget to rehydrate with water or a sports drink after your run. If your urine is dark yellow after your run, you need to keep rehydrating. It should be a light lemonade color.

Staying well-hydrated will help prevent muscle cramps, but if you're dealing with cramps on a run, try slowly stretching the affected area. Stopping to stretch for a minute or two during a run will help keep the cramps from getting worse.

A sports massage is a good way to treat soreness that often develops as a result of muscle cramps. Regular massages also help keep your muscles in optimal shape, greatly reducing your chances of muscle cramping during runs.

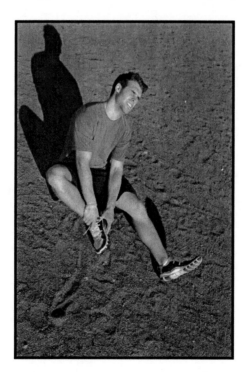

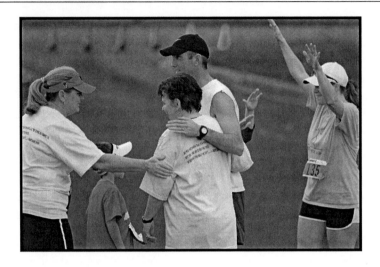

Despite your best injury prevention efforts, you may find yourself dealing with some aches and pains. Most running injuries take a few weeks to develop and then another couple of weeks to heal. Learn more about these common running injuries, their causes, and treatments.

Achilles Tendonitis

Achilles tendonitis is an injury that occurs when your Achilles tendon—the large band of tissues connecting the muscles in the back of your lower leg to your heel bone—becomes inflamed or irritated.

Ankle Sprains

Ankle sprains are often caused by the twisting or rolling of your ankle, resulting in swelling and pain above and around the ankle.

Black Toenails

Runners, especially those training for long-distance events, can suffer from black toenails, caused by the toes rubbing up against the front of the running shoe. A blood blister forms under the toenail and the nail eventually falls off.

Blisters

While not a serious injury, blisters—those fluid-filled bubbles of skin on your feet—can be painful and keep you from running.

Illiotibial Band Syndrome

Marked by a sharp, burning knee or hip pain, Illiotibial Band Syndrome (ITBS) is a very common injury among runners.

Muscle Pulls or Strains

Muscle pulls and strains are common and annoying injuries for runners, marked by pain and tightness in the affected muscle.

Runner's Knee

A common complaint among long-distance runners, runner's knee feels like a soreness around and sometimes behind the kneecap.

Plantar Fasciitis

Heel pain in runners is usually caused by inflammation of the plantar fascia, a condition known as plantar fasciitis.

Shin Splints

One of the most common injuries for beginner runners, shin splints are characterized by pain in the front of the lower leg.

Stress Fractures

Stress fractures, or tiny cracks in the surface of a bone, are serious running injuries that requires immediate treatment.

By Christine Luff, www.running.about.com

Questions?

_____

_____

_____

_____

_____

_____

_____

Week 5 Workout Plan

Workout 1, 2, and 3

    Brisk 5-minute warm-up walk

    Jog 3 minutes

    Walk 90 seconds

    Jog 5 minutes

    Walk 2 minutes

    Jog 3 minutes

    Walk 90 seconds

    Jog 5 minutes

    Walk 3 minutes

    <u>5-minute cool-down walk</u>

    Total Workout = 34 Minutes

Break it Down

Instead of always asking God for what you want, try asking for a better understanding of what he wants. Often we are simply asking the wrong questions.

Tip of the Week

Listen Up!

"You must listen to your body. Run through annoyance, but not through pain."

—*Dr. George Shaheen*

Week 6: If you Have to Ask ...

Story

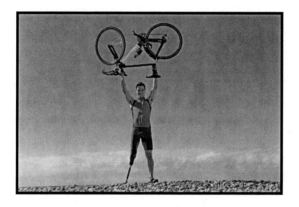

"... And ye shall know the truth, and the truth shall make you free."

—John 8:32 (KJV)

I have a patch with the Ironman Triathlon symbol in the center. Around the outside it reads, "If you have to ask, you wouldn't understand." There's a certain truth to that statement. I know; I've asked. I did one, and now I know. But it is something you can't understand until you have been there and had a chance to look at it from the other side of the mirror, so to speak.

This concept applies to more than just Ironman Triathlons. Last Saturday, as I leaned forward into 30 to 50 mph winds on a training run, I pondered how similar endurance training is to a relationship with Jesus. There's a depth of experiencing Him that comes only as a result of having endured—regardless of the weather, regardless of pain, regardless of people's glances, whispers, and snide remarks. For me, it has come about slowly, through the wrestling matches I've had with Him over the years and in the moments of peace in between. In quiet reflection, I can see that I've experienced Him when we've been locked together in the fiercest of battles. Yet, at the end of each, when I finally submitted to Him and stopped struggling, I found myself experiencing the most powerful and loving embrace I've ever known. I've held long, lopsided discussions with Him on lonely running trails. In response, He's woven His replies into the fabric of my life in different ways and at different times.

We are different; we are endurance athletes. There are those who don't understand us. In much the same way, we are different; we are followers of Christ. There are many who don't understand us. There are many who insult and despise us. But endure, my friend. The experience of truth is well worth the battle. Jesus said He is the Truth, and, "you will know the truth, and the truth will set you free ..."

Story by Donna Douglass, www.donnadouglass.com

Discussion

Have you experienced God in your life?

_____

_____

_____

Have you stepped aside from the busyness of life to reflect on what God is doing in and around you?

_____

_____

_____

Do you listen for His voice in His Word, and then watch for His promises to manifest in your life?

_____

_____

_____

How can you help someone else experience God?

_____

_____

_____

*G*et in the Word

Workout 1—Isaiah 55:8–9

_____

_____

_____

Workout 2—John 8:32

_____

_____

_____

Workout 3—John 14:6

_____

_____

_____

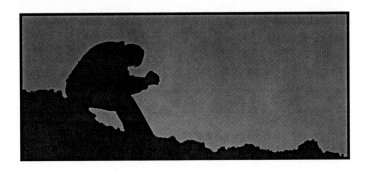

_____

_____

_____

_____

_____

_____

_____

_____

*B*asic Nutrition

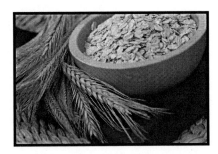

As a runner, your diet is important not only for maintaining good health, but also to promote peak performance. Proper nutrition and hydration can make or break a workout or race, and it also greatly affects how runners feel, work, and think.

A balanced diet for healthy runners should include these essentials: carbohydrates, protein, fats, vitamins, and minerals. Here are some basic guidelines for a nutritious, healthy balance.

Carbohydrates

Carbohydrates should make up about 60 percent of a runner's total calorie intake. Without a doubt, carbs are the best source of energy for athletes. Research has shown that for both quick and long-lasting energy, our bodies work more efficiently with carbs than they do with proteins or fats. Whole grain pasta, steamed or boiled rice, potatoes, fruits, starchy vegetables, and whole grain breads are good carb sources.

Protein

Protein is used for some energy and to repair tissue damaged during training. Protein should make up about 15 to 20 percent of your daily intake. Runners, especially those running long distances, should consume .5 to .75 grams of protein per pound of body weight. Try to concentrate on protein sources that are low in fat and cholesterol such as lean meats, fish, low-fat dairy products, poultry, whole grains, and beans.

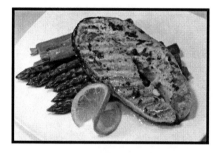

Fat

A high fat diet can quickly pack on the pounds, so try to make sure that no more than 20 to 25 percent of your total diet comes from fats. Stick to foods low in saturated fats and cholesterol. Foods such as nuts, oils, and cold-water fish provide essential fats called omega–3s, which are vital for good health and can help prevent certain diseases. Most experts recommend getting about 3,000 mg of omega–3 fat a day.

Vitamins

Runners don't get energy from vitamins, but they are still an important part of their diet. Exercise may produce compounds called free radicals, which can damage cells. Vitamins C, E, and A are antioxidants and can neutralize free radicals. Getting your vitamins from whole foods is preferable to supplementation; there's no strong evidence that taking supplements improves either health or athletic performance.

𝓜inerals

Calcium: A calcium-rich diet is essential for runners to prevent osteoporosis and stress fractures. Good sources of calcium include low-fat dairy products, calcium-fortified juices, dark leafy vegetables, beans, and eggs. Your goal should be 1,000 to 1,300 mg of calcium per day.

Iron: You need this nutrient to deliver oxygen to your cells. If you have an iron-poor diet, you'll feel weak and fatigued, especially when you run. Men should aim for 8 mg of iron a day, and women need 18 mg. Good natural sources of iron include lean meats, leafy green vegetables, nuts, shrimp, and scallops.

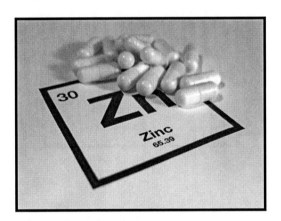

Sodium and other electrolytes: Small amounts of sodium and other electrolytes are lost through sweat during exercise. Usually, electrolytes are replaced if you follow a balanced diet. But if you find yourself craving salty foods, it may be your body's way of telling you to get more sodium. Try drinking a sports drink or eating some pretzels after exercise.

By Christine Luff, www.running.about.com

Questions?

_____

_____

_____

_____

_____

_____

_____

_____

Week 6 Workout Plan

Workout 1, 2, and 3

    Brisk 5-minute warm-up walk

    Jog 3 minutes

    Walk 90 seconds

    Jog 5 minutes

    Walk 2 minutes

    Jog 3 minutes

    Walk 90 seconds

    Jog 5 minutes

    Walk 3 minutes

    5-minute cool-down walk

    Total Workout = 34 Minutes

Break it Down

The title of the story above is "If you have to ask." We must acknowledge that if someone is asking about our faith, chances are that they do not understand, and it is our job to help them get there.

Tip of the Week

Reflect ...

"After finishing a run take a minute and look back at where you came from, ahead at where you are going, and thank God for the opportunity."

—*Mitchell Hollis*, **Run For God**

Week 7: Starving the Rabbit

Story

> "As His divine power has given to us all things that *pertain* to life and godliness, through the knowledge of Him who called us by glory and virtue, 4 by which have been given to us exceedingly great and precious promises, that through these you may be partakers of the divine nature, having escaped the corruption *that is* in the world through lust."
>
> —2 Peter 1:3–4 (NKJV)

It was just a matter of time. But even though it was inevitable, we saw it coming. My kids had had a pet rabbit for many years. They loved the rabbit and took great care of it. However, over the years, as activities increased and life got busier for three growing children, it become difficult for them to find time to feed the rabbit. I covered for them occasionally, but the rabbit simply did not get the food it needed. One day we went to the cage to find a motionless rabbit. It had died. The kids didn't mean to starve it, or even want to see their pet die. But when you don't feed a rabbit, it dies.

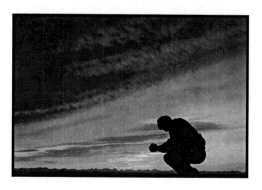

It was a tough example to learn from. Life lessons hurt. I was mad, the kids were crushed, and the rabbit was dead. The lesson of this story is that when you stop doing the things you need to do, destructive results are inevitable. As I thought about the mistake of my kids, the Lord actually convicted me. (I hate it when the Lord starts shining the spotlight on me when I want it to shine on someone else.) But in my spirit, the Lord said, "Dan, you do the same thing. You know you should feed your soul with the Word of God. When you don't, you starve me, because my Spirit lives inside of you." Ouch!

My children didn't want to starve the rabbit. In the same way, I don't want to starve the living God who dwells in me. But when I don't carve out the daily time for Him, I starve Him. We need to make sure that the busyness of life doesn't crowd out, squeeze out, or starve out Jesus. You care about Jesus. You love Jesus. Maybe you just don't care enough to be spiritually healthy and you allow yourself to become spiritually malnourished. You eat just enough to get by, taking in a short devotional here and there or having a quick word of prayer so that God can bless something you are doing. You just skim when it comes to the things of God. After all, compared to all your friends, you are doing great! (Probably because they are doing nothing.) Other people replace God as your standard.

What you do for your spiritual health you would never do for your physical health. Not many of us are missing meals. But many of us are missing our spiritual meals. When you see the pictures of children in Africa starving to death, your heart breaks for them. Maybe God looks at us in the same way. Maybe He sees us like a starving, malnourished child, barely alive spiritually, and His heart breaks. Only you and the Lord know if you are spiritually well fed and healthy or if you are starving to death.

As competitors, we understand the importance of physical health. If we don't take care of our bodies and train, we pay the price. But Jesus wants us to take care of our souls and train spiritually so that we will be ready and prepared as warriors of God for whatever the gates of hell throw at us. If we are spiritually weak, we will be crushed. If we are spiritually strong, the life of Christ will be manifested through us and bring victory!

Today, do something that only you can do. Get spiritually healthy. I think you know what you need to do. Pray, read, study, meditate, share, fellowship, memorize. Do whatever it takes to get healthy. Your future depends on it. And your Lord and Savior is waiting.

Story by Dan Britton, FCA

_____

_____

_____

_____

_____

_____

_____

_____

*D*iscussion

1. How is your soul doing? Are you healthy spiritually? Are you missing spiritual meals? _____

_____

_____

2. Why are you in your current spiritual condition? What has brought you to this point? What excuses or compromises have you made that left you spiritually malnourished? What disciplines have you put in place that have made you spiritually strong? _____

_____

_____

_____

3. What can you do today that will help you get healthy? Commit to this answer for thirty days. Seek accountability from a trusted friend. _____

_____

_____

_____

*G*et in the Word

Workout 1—Mark 1:35

_____

_____

_____

Workout 2—2 Peter 1:3–11

_____

_____

_____

Workout 3—2 Timothy 4:7–8

_____

_____

_____

_____

*C*ommon Weight Loss Mistakes

Mistake 1: Unrealistic Expectations

While television shows such as *The Biggest Loser* may inspire people to lose weight, they also set them up for very unrealistic weight-loss expectations. Just because someone on TV loses ten pounds in a week doesn't mean that it's safe, healthy, or realistic for you to do the same thing.

How to fix it: A healthy amount of weight loss is a pound to two pounds per week. Research shows that people who lose a lot of weight very quickly are more likely to gain it back. (Just as you may have seen in the "Where Are They Now?" episodes of those weight loss shows.) It's important to be patient and see each lost pound to be a huge achievement along the way. Remember to have ways other than the number on the scale to measure your progress, such as how your clothes fit or the number of inches you've lost. Think about all the other healthy improvements you're seeing, including reduced stress, improved sleep, increased energy, and reduced risk of many diseases.

Mistake 2: Depriving Yourself

You may assume that being on a diet or eating healthy means giving up all your favorite indulgent foods. But what happens if you deprive yourself too much is that it usually leads to overeating. One day you just cave in and then you really go overboard.

How to fix it: If you have a really strong craving, it's fine to indulge—a little. Try to prevent yourself from going overboard by placing only a certain amount of food in front of you. Put potato chips in a small bowl rather than eating them right out of the bag, for example. This is especially important after a tough run or workout, when you may feel that a big-calorie binge is justified. In reality, you could end up eating way more calories than you burned during your run.

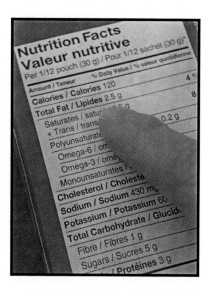

Mistake 3: Using Food as a Reward

Whether they're trying to lose weight or not, it's very common for runners to use food as a reward. They often want to treat themselves after a hard workout or race. But that kind of reward system can really derail your weight-loss efforts. You may start using every little excuse to treat yourself to a high-calorie dessert or other indulgence when you have an urge for it.

How to fix it: Instead, treat yourself to non-food rewards, such as new running gear or a massage when you reach a running goal.

Mistake 4: Skipping Meals

Some people skip meals thinking that they'll save calories. But that strategy usually backfires. Our bodies have a built-in survival mechanism to conserve calories when we go for a long time without eating. When you skip meals, your body slows your metabolism to prevent you from starving. Skipping a meal will make you hungrier, which increases your temptation to eat everything in sight.

How to Fix It: Try to eat five to six small meals each day, or three meals and some healthy snacks in between. You'll find that eating mini meals will help maintain your energy levels throughout the day and keep you from feeling hungry (and then binging) all the time. If you skip meals such as breakfast because you don't have time, try eating something quick like cereal, peanut butter on toast, or cottage cheese and fruit.

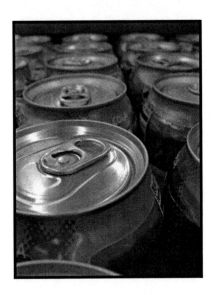

Mistake 5: Drinking Too Many Calories

Some runners assume that because they're running or doing other forms of exercise, they're supposed to drink sports drinks. But the truth is that, while it's important that you use sports drinks to replace electrolytes during your long runs, you don't need to constantly drink them when you're not running. Not only are they high in calories, but they also have very little nutritional benefit and they won't keep you full.

How to fix it: Stay away from sugary sports drinks, unless you're running more than 90 minutes and need to replace electrolytes lost through sweat. You should also try to avoid fruit juices (whole fruit is always better), regular soda, and high-calorie specialty coffee beverages. Plain water is fine for staying hydrated during the week. If that's too boring for you, try squeezing a lemon in your water or drink no-calorie flavored seltzer water.

Mistake 6: Overestimating Your Calories Burned

Some people trying to lose weight will rely on calorie expenditure tables to figure out how many calories they're burning while running or doing other physical activities. The problem is that those tables tell you the calorie expenditure of an average person and usually overestimate the calorie expenditure. The same is true for treadmills and other cardio machines that display calorie expenditures. Some reports suggest that treadmills and other cardio machines actually overestimate calories burned by up to 15 to 20 percent.

How to fix it: It's important that you take calories burned estimates with a grain of salt. It's fine to use the numbers as a benchmark for your runs, but don't plan on consuming additional calories based on that number. That's an easy way to start gaining weight, despite your exercise efforts. If you really want to get a better idea of how many calories you're burning during your runs, try using a heart rate monitor. That will be more accurate than relying on tables or cardio machine readings.

Mistake 7: Not Readjusting Calorie Needs

As you lose weight, your calorie needs change because it takes fewer calories to maintain your weight. If you keep eating the same amount of calories, you'll probably hit a weight loss plateau.

How to fix it: If you want to keep losing weight, you have to gradually reduce your calorie intake.

By Christine Luff, www.running.about.com

Questions?

_____

_____

_____

_____

*W*eek 7 Workout Plan

Workout 1

    Brisk 5-minute warm-up walk

    Jog 5 minutes

    Walk 3 minutes

    Jog 5 minutes

    Walk 3 minutes

    Jog 5 minutes

    <u>5-minute cool-down walk</u>

    Total Workout = 31 Minutes

Workouts 2 & 3

    Brisk 5-minute warm-up walk

    Jog 8 minutes

    Walk 5 minutes

    Jog 8 minutes

    <u>5-minute cool-down walk</u>

    Total Workout = 31 Minutes

*B*reak it Down

Make time every day for the Lord even if it means sacrificing something else that you love—it will be well worth the sacrifice!

Tip of The Week

Stick to your plan ...

By now you may be getting comfortable with the exercises and feel that you need to skip ahead. Beware; this can lead to injuries that will only cause frustration and regret.

Week 8: Yes, you can!

$\mathcal{R}$ead It

"I can do all things through Christ which strengtheneth me."

9—Philippians 4:13 (KJV)

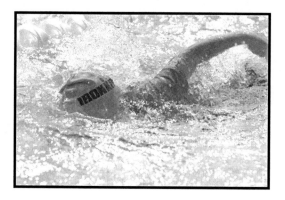

I can remember signing my son Lane up for his very first Iron Kids triathlon. He was six years old and extremely excited that he was actually going to get to compete in his very own triathlon. There was one problem, however; Lane was at best a decent doggy paddler and in just a few months he would have to cover 50 meters in an Olympic size pool. Right now he could barely cover 10 feet.

I can remember the first time that I got Lane into the pool at our local gym. He was all but terrified at the thought of having to swim from one end of the pool to the other, and that was only 25 meters. He would grab my neck and say, "I can't, Daddy, I can't." I would have to explain to him that all I wanted for him to do was try, because I knew he could. I would assure him that I was not going to let anything happen to him and that he was safe because I was there with him. It was not long before Lane really got the hang of swimming and he finally understood that if he listened to what his father was saying, everything would be fine.

How many times do we as Christians do the very same thing with Jesus? We sense that we are being called to do something, whether it is to serve more in our church or to reach out and witness to an individual. We plead with God, telling him we can't—sound familiar? We have every excuse under the sun and none of them are good. We expect our children to listen and understand that we know what is best, but why is it so difficult for us to trust God and do what he says? He always knows what's best, he will always be with you, anything is possible through him, and he is always just a prayer away.

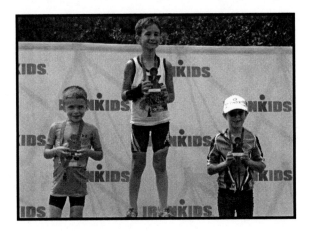

Oh, and by the way. Lane did finish his first Iron Kids event. He placed second in his age group at the Alpharetta, Georgia, Iron Kids.

By Mitchell Hollis

Discussion

Why is our answer too often "I can't" when the Lord asks something of us?

_____

_____

_____

_____

How does it feel when you push through the "I can't" and you finish with an "I did?" _____

_____

_____

_____

_____

𝒢et in the Word

Workout 1—Philippians 4:13

_____

_____

_____

Workout 2—Romans 8:35–39

_____

_____

_____

Workout 3—Hebrews 11:1

_____

_____

_____

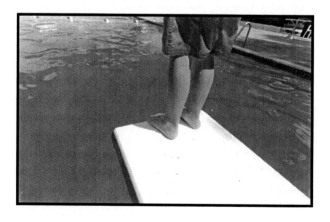

Staying Motivated

Staying motivated to run is one of the problems facing many runners. Whether you are a novice runner or a runner who has been running for years, it can be difficult to stay motivated to run on a regular basis. A number of factors may contribute to a loss of motivation. Some of these factors may include boredom, muscle soreness, or even a lack of time. If you are like most runners, you have likely faced a lack of motivation at least once in your running career. It may start out slowly, with you skipping one or two runs here and there, but it may gradually progress to the point where you are rarely running. This article will provide a number of tips for keeping a runner motivated to stick with a running program.

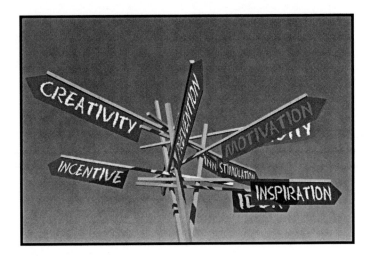

Setting realistic goals is one of the easiest ways for a runner to stay motivated to continue running. One of the common goals runners like to use to stay motivated is a goal of completing a race. Selecting a race and training for and competing in the event can provide a great source of motivation, which can prevent a runner from abandoning a running program. You may select a long distance event such as a marathon or shorter events such as a 10K race, a 5K race, or even shorter events. The distance of the event you select should depend on your personal goals. If you simply want to stay motivated to run on a regular basis, competing in short races periodically is an excellent way to stay on track. Setting such a goal is motivating because the runner is capable of focusing on the training.

Another goal a runner may wish to set is to improve race times on a regular basis. For example, a runner who recently completed a 5K race in 35 minutes may set a goal of completing a subsequent 5K race in a faster time of approximately 33 minutes. With this goal in mind, the runner will likely stay motivated to continue running so they can achieve the goal when he or she enters the next race. Runners can then continue to set progressively faster goals or may branch out and set goals of running longer races once they reach a point where they feel as though they cannot improve on their speed anymore.

Runners can also stay motivated to keep up a running program by incorporating variety. Many runners make the mistake of running laps on a track or following the same course through their neighborhood every time. They think this is the only way to stay dedicated. However, this couldn't be farther from the truth. This mentality can lead to both mental and physical burnout. Additionally, the runner will not likely improve under this type of program because the body will become more efficient at completing the course and, as a result, will require fewer calories and will tax the muscles less in completing the course. A better approach to running is to vary the courses in terms of distance, speed, intensity, and terrain regularly to keep both the mind and the body challenged.

These variations in a workout are relatively easy to incorporate but can be very effective for keeping the workouts interesting. The terrain can be varied by running on trails that have a series of hills. This change of pace will likely make the surroundings more interesting and the varied terrain will challenge the runner's body in new ways. Runners can vary the intensity of a workout by incorporating sprint intervals into the running. A runner who regularly runs four miles on a track can modify his workout a few days a week by sprinting on the straight sections of the track and jogging on the curved portions. These sprint intervals make the workout seem to go faster, and challenge the muscles in a different way.

Running with a friend is another way for a runner to stick with a running program. Running does not have to be a solitary activity. Having a friend along can not only keep you motivated but can also make the runs more enjoyable. You can chat with your friend about a number of different subjects to pass the time, which will make the running seem less monotonous. You can also challenge each other to improve by having friendly competitions. Another reason running with a partner helps a runner to stay motivated is that most people are likely to fulfill their obligations when someone else is counting on them. Sometimes just knowing someone is waiting to run with you can motivate you to complete your workout. Conversely, if you are working out alone, it is much easier to decide to take the day off.

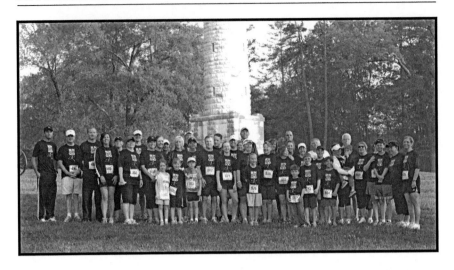

Finally, it is important for runners to take some time off from running occasionally. This may sound counterintuitive, but it is actually quite effective. Cross training can help a runner stay in shape but can also give him a well deserved break from running. One way to incorporate cross training into your running program is to participate in another type of activity in place of your running one or two days per week. For example, you may wish to ride a bike on these days instead of running. Another day to incorporate cross training into your workout routine is to take one week every couple of months where you don't run at all but you engage in other physical activities. After your brief hiatus from running, you will likely find yourself recharged and less likely to give up your running program all together.

By www.therunnersguide.com

_____

_____

_____

_____

_____

_____

_____

_____

_____

Questions?

_____

_____

_____

_____

_____

_____

_____

_____

Week 8 Workout Plan

Workout 1, 2, & 3

    Brisk 5-minute warm-up walk

    Jog 20 minutes

    5-minute cool-down walk

    Total Workout = 30 Minutes

Week 8 Conclusion

We often doubt if what we are thinking is really what the Lord is saying. Pray that the Lord will make his requests like a flashing neon sign, easy to see and follow, and remember that the more time you spend with the Lord, the easier his voice is to recognize.

Tip of The Week

    "Whether you believe you can or believe you can't, you're probably right."

—Henry Ford

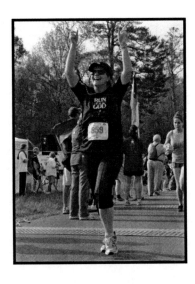

Week 9: The Right Race

Story

> "Therefore we also, since we are surrounded by so great a cloud of witnesses, let us lay aside every weight, and the sin which so easily ensnares *us*, and let us run with endurance the race that is set before us."
>
> —Hebrews 12:1 (NKJV)

The first race I ever ran was a marathon, an incredible experience my body will never forget. I learned there are four key aspects to a race, and they all relate to our spiritual life.

We race against competition. There were thousands of runners I wanted to beat and who wanted to beat me. When we run the race for Christ, we compete against the world, the flesh, and the Devil. We race against the clock. Every mile I clocked declared I was nearing the end. People say since we only go around once, live it up. Christ says since we only go around once, make it count.

We race for a prize. I received a medal for completing the marathon. As Christians, our prize is heaven and eternity with God!

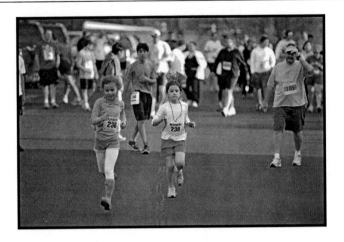

We race for praise. It was awesome to have hundreds of people cheering as I crossed the finish line, but it won't compare to hearing Christ say, "Well done, good and faithful servant."

Are you running the right race or the rat race? If we win the rat race, we are still a rat. The rat race gets our eyes off Christ—it is the wrong race. Run the right race—the race of Christ.

Story by Dan Britton, FCA

*D*iscussion

What race are you running? _____

_____

_____

Which of the three competitors do you battle most? _____

_____

_____

What needs to happen in your life for you to run the right race? _____

_____

_____

$\mathcal{G}$et in the Word

Workout 1—1 Corinthians 9:24–26

Workout 2—Philippians 2:14–16

Workout 3—Romans 6:11

$\mathcal{M}$uscle vs. Fat

Is muscle heavier than fat? It's a weighty question.

Providing a quick answer to the "which weighs more?" question can be misleading, as it all depends on what the question is really about.

There may, indeed be a short-term weight gain when you begin an exercise program. Of course, a pound of muscle weighs exactly the same as a pound of fat. Fat, however, is slightly less dense than muscle, meaning that a set volume of muscle will weigh slightly more than the same volume of fat.

The core of the confusion about this relates to the difference between weight and caloric density, which is the number of calories per unit of weight. The calorie is a unit of energy in the body. A gram of fat has more than twice the calories of a gram of protein or a gram of carbohydrate.

For an analogy, consider the dollar as a unit of spending energy. A $10 bill weighs exactly the same as a $5 bill. But there is a difference in their spending density, the monetary value per unit of weight. Using our definition, a $10 bill would have twice the spending density of a $5 bill.

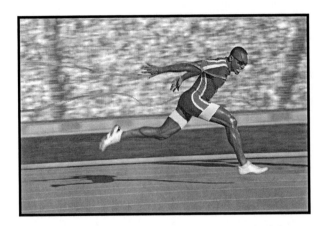

Humans are water-based organisms, and most of what goes on metabolically involves transport through a water-based medium. Fat, which is the most concentrated form of energy in the human body, is the way the body stores its energy. Adipose tissue, which is where our fat is stored, is not very active metabolically, and it contains very little water.

By contrast, the protein that makes up our metabolically active muscles and organs is mostly water.

The body does not like to waste energy, so it only keeps the amount of muscle needed to maintain the status quo. Extra muscle means more energy being burned, even while at rest. Think about an 8-cylinder engine burning gas at idle, versus a 4-cylinder engine at the same speed.

If we become less active, the body slowly reduces its muscular mass down to that needed to keep the show going. When we pick up the pace, the body responds by building more muscle.

During exercise, our energy demands are primarily fueled by body fat. Exercise is a stress on a body that is not used to a workout. The stress extends to the muscles as well as the heart and circulatory system. If the energy demand becomes routine, the body reduces the stress by building new muscles to handle the load and by increasing blood volume to carry the nutrients and waste products, and lung capacity to deliver oxygen (and remove carbon dioxide) as needed.

Let's assume you are eating a fixed number of calories and begin your exercise program. As you make new muscles and other supporting tissues, you call on your energy-dense tissue (adipose) to create new muscle and other tissues that are primarily water.

The numbers on the scale will go up slightly, but it is important to realize that you are mostly gaining water weight. You are not getting fatter, but home scales do not provide that breakdown.

If you were to stop exercising, you might actually lose weight. But, again, you are losing water, and you might be getting fatter at the same time. Focusing solely on the numbers on the scale can be discouraging because it does not give you the complete picture, even when good things are going on inside.

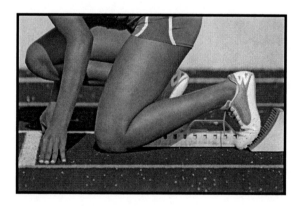

Becoming more fit is a good thing. It enhances your body's ability to handle stress, and you create metabolically active tissue that will burn calories even when you are sitting around reading a book. Making it a habit is an important part of the picture; otherwise, you will lose that stress-coping, calorie-burning advantage.

By Ed Blonz, PHD

Questions?

_____

_____

_____

_____

_____

_____

_____

_____

Week 9 Workout Plan

Workouts 1, 2, & 3

Brisk 5-minute warm-up walk

Jog 23 minutes

5-minute cool-down walk

Total Workout = 33 Minutes

Break it Down

Don't lose focus of your goal, whether that goal be physical, mental, or spiritual. Keep your eye on the goal and don't complain about the hurdles you have to jump in getting there.

Tip of the Week

"**Heaven** … All that matters is that you get there. Speed is irrelevant."

—*Mitchell Hollis,* **Run for God**

Week 10: Pancakes/Waffles

Remember to order your Race Day shirts!

*R*ead It

> "Set your mind on things above, not on things on the earth."
>
> —Colossians 3:2 (NKJV)

Are you a pancake or waffle? This question was posed to me in my Sunday School class one morning. The class was discussing the differences between the two. We are often like waffles in that we try to fit time with God into a compartment, much like syrup fits into the little holes on a waffle, instead of covering our lives with God like syrup on a pancake. We didn't stay on this topic for very long before we moved on.

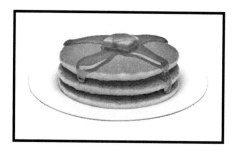

The next topic was time and how we manage it. Most everyone in our class has young children and people were sharing how ball games, dance, school, work, and many other things just take away their time. All of us find ourselves at the end of the week with no time left for God. This discussion immediately took me back to the pancake/waffle analogy.

Not even ten minutes earlier, our class had been discussing the pitfalls of living our faith lives like waffles, and now we were complaining about not having the time for God—might that be the compartment for God? I began to realize that this is just an accepted state of mind in our culture. Everything has its place and you should not let one thing in your life affect the other things. Really, there is nothing wrong with this train of thought—not until you factor in your faith.

This got me to thinking about the reason that I started Run For God. You see, endurance sports had began to fill my life and had slowly squeezed out my "Christian Life Compartment." I was convicted not of my love for running, but of not including God in the things that I love. God does not ask us to stop doing the things we love, but rather asks us to use these things to glorify him and to further his kingdom. It doesn't matter if you are at a T-Ball game, playing golf, shopping, or driving down the road, you CAN glorify God in almost everything you do. We just have to learn to live like pancakes and let God's love and direction flood every "compartment" of our lives.

By Mitchell Hollis

Discussion

Are you living your life like a pancake or waffle? _____

_____

_____

_____

_____

_____

How can you include the things that you love into God's plan for your life? _____

_____

_____

_____

If you are doing something that does not glorify God, is it a sin? __

_____

_____

_____

_____

_____

_____

_____

_____

_____

*G*et in the Word

Workout 1—1 Corinthians 10:14

_____

_____

_____

Workout 2—1 Corinthians 12:4–6

_____

_____

_____

Workout 3—Colossians 3:17

_____

_____

_____

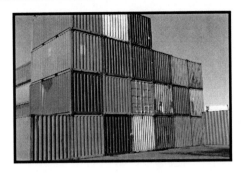

$\mathcal{R}$oad Race Etiquette

If you're new to running in road races, you may not be familiar with some of the rules—both stated and unwritten. While many veteran runners love to see new runners joining the sport, they have pet peeves about inconsiderate behavior from other runners, especially beginners. To avoid annoying fellow runners (and prevent looking like a newbie), be sure to follow these etiquette guidelines when participating in races:

Pay for Your Spot

Running in a race you haven't entered, also called "banditting," is not fair to race organizers, volunteers, and especially the people who have paid to participate. It's also unsafe, since race organizers plan their course amenities, such as water and sports drinks and medical assistance based on the number of people who have signed up for the race. Overcrowded race conditions can lead to falls and other problems.

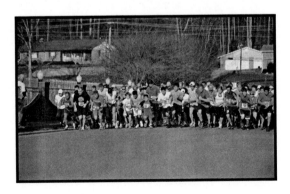

Line Up Properly

Nothing is more annoying to a runner at the start of a race than having to weave around slower runners after the gun goes off. Faster runners should line up at the front of the starting line, slower runners and walkers at the back. Some races have corrals based on estimated pace or post pace signs. If not, ask runners nearby their anticipated pace, and if it's faster than yours, move further back. Most races use timing chips, so the time it takes you to reach the starting line won't count in your final net time.

Don't Jingle

Don't carry loose change or a set of keys in your pocket. They'll annoy those who are running near you.

Don't Take Up the Whole Road

If you're running with a group, try not to run more than two abreast, so others can pass you.

Show Appreciation to Volunteers

Say thank you to race volunteers who hand you water or put your medal around your neck. They're volunteering their time, and the race would not be successful without them.

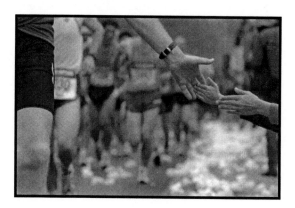

Thank Supporters, Too

Acknowledge supporters who cheer for you as you pass them. If you're too tired to say thanks, show them a smile, wave, or give them a thumbs up. It will make them feel good and encourage them to keep rooting for others.

Be Careful at Water Stations

Water stations can get a bit chaotic and crowded. Use caution when running into a water stop and make sure you're not cutting off other runners or spilling water on them. If you're going to stop or slow down to walk through the water stop, make sure there's not a runner behind you.

Keep Moving at the Finish

Don't immediately stop at the finish line or in the chute. There will be runners coming in right behind you, so keep going until it's safe to come to a stop.

Don't Be a Glutton

Don't take more than your fair share of food and drinks at the finish line. The back of the pack runners will appreciate it when there are still enough goodies for them at the end.

By Christine Luff, www.running.about.com

_____

_____

_____

_____

_____

Questions?

_____

_____

_____

_____

_____

_____

Week 10 Workout Plan

Workouts 1, 2, & 3

Brisk 5-minute warm-up walk

Jog 27 minutes

5-minute cool-down walk

Total Workout = 37 Minutes

Week 10 Conclusion

If you don't already, begin including God in everything that you do. Many people choose to have a partner to run with. They share the ups and downs of the sport together and really form a close bond with one another. Ask God to be your running partner as well!

Tip of the Week

Idol ... Don't let anything become your idol!

Week 11: Know your MP3

$\mathcal{S}$tory

> "Keep thy tongue from evil, and thy lips from speaking guile."
>
> —Psalms 34:13 (KJV)

Over the past several years a new toy has exploded in the running world as a must have for your gear bag. I am talking about the MP3 player. These devices have revolutionized the music industry. What once took a very large piece of equipment to store hours and hours of music has now been reduced to half the size of a credit card. You can have all your favorite music organized any way you want it, and all at the touch of a button. The sound is great, they weigh only ounces, and you don't even notice ear plugs in your ears.

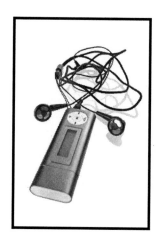

MP3s have become a great tool for runners, but they can also become a distraction from your spiritual life. You see I used to have music on my MP3 player that I normally would not listen to if I were not exercising. Experts say that the best exercise music is 90 beats per minute (BPM), and for a southern gospel fan like me this was hard to find. I began putting secular music of the worst kind on my MP3. I justified this by telling myself that I was only doing it for the tempo and that I just would not pay any attention to the lyrics. A disturbing thing began to happen. I would find myself singing along to these songs not only while running, but also when I heard those songs out in public.

Everything in this world has the potential to influence us, even the music that we listen to. We have all seen the WWJD bracelets (what would Jesus do). That is a great question to keep in our minds at all times. If Jesus were walking the streets today listening to his MP3, would he have a playlist like I did? I think we all know the answer to this question, which brings up another question. What music do you have on your playlist?

By Mitchell Hollis

_____

_____

_____

_____

_____

_____

_____

_____

*D*iscussion

How does music affect your walk with God? _____

_____

_____

Would you be comfortable with your pastor listening to your MP3? _____

_____

_____

_____

*S*tudy It

Workout 1—Deuteronomy 6:5

_____

_____

_____

Workout 2—1 John 3:2–3

_____

_____

_____

Workout 3—1 Corinthians 10:31

_____

_____

_____

*T*he Best Foods For Runners

1. Whole Grain Pasta and Bread

Why they're good for runners: Runners need plenty of carbohydrates to fuel workouts, and breads and pasta are obvious choices. But, let's face it, not all bread and pasta is created equal. Whole grain foods are less processed and therefore contain more of the natural nutrition found in the grain, including more fiber. Compared to white pasta and bread, you'll get more nutrients from whole grains, and the increased fiber will help you feel fuller longer.

How to add it to your diet: Stock up on whole-grain breads, pasta, rolls, crackers, and cereal. Try to avoid white bread or any baked products made with white flour.

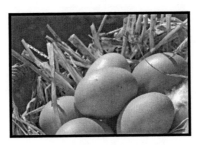

2. Eggs

Why they're good for runners: One egg satisfies about 10 percent of your daily protein needs, and the amino acids in eggs will help with muscle repair and recovery. You'll also get about 30 percent of your recommended amount of vitamin K, which is crucial for bone health.

How to add them to your diet: Whether you like them boiled, scrambled, poached, or fried, eggs can be eaten anytime of the day. Mix up your routine by having an omelet or frittata for dinner.

_____

_____

_____

_____

_____

_____

_____

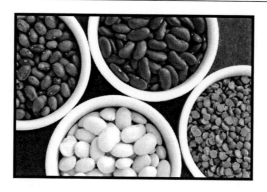

3. Beans

Why they're good for runners: Cooked dry beans like pinto, lentil, garbanzo, and split pea are high in protein and fiber, a plant source of iron and low in fat.

How to add them to your diet: Beans are a great accompaniment to soups and stews. Rice and beans makes an easy meal that contains both carbs and protein.

4. Salmon

Why it's good for runners: Salmon is an excellent protein source, but it's also one of the best food sources of omega–3 fats, essential for brain development and function. Omega–3s also assist in the prevention of heart disease and high blood pressure. Salmon also has protein, vitamins A, B, and D as well as a range of minerals vital to a balanced and healthy diet.

How to add it to your diet: Salmon is a very versatile fish—just add some fresh herbs and bake, grill, or poach it. Even canned salmon is good for you. It can be used in salads, sandwiches, and chowder.

5. Sweet Potatoes

Why they're good for runners: Sweet potatoes contain the always-important carbs and are an excellent source vitamin A, a powerful antioxidant. They're also a good source of vitamin C, potassium, and iron.

How to add them to your diet: As the name says, these potatoes are sweet, so you don't need to do much to make them taste good. Cook them in the microwave, add a pinch of margarine or butter, and you've got a great side for dinner. Or slice them up into wedges and bake some tasty oven fries.

6. Low-Fat Yogurt

Why it's good for runners: Low-fat yogurt is a great source protein and carbs. It also contains calcium, which is important for runners, especially those at risk for stress fractures.

How to add it to your diet: Eat a container of low-fat yogurt as a mid-morning or mid-afternoon snack or make tasty smoothies with yogurt, ice, and your favorite fresh or frozen fruits.

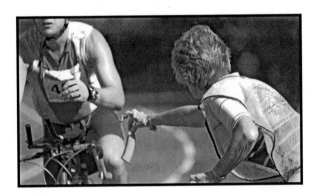

7. Bananas

Why they're good for runners: A good source of carbs, bananas also contain potassium, which runners lose through sweating. The fruit also help regulate muscle contraction and prevent cramping. Bananas are also considered a "safe" pre-run food because they're unlikely to cause gastrointestinal issues.

How to add them to your diet: Bananas are convenient to eat as snacks or as part of a meal. Add them to your cereal or make a smoothie with frozen bananas and skim milk.

8. Peanut Butter

Why it's good for runners: Peanut butter is tasty and satisfying, which makes it a great food for runners who are trying to lose weight. The protein and fiber in peanut butter helps you feel full and it's not fattening, unless you overeat total calories that day. For example, eating a whole-wheat bagel with peanut butter will make you feel fuller than if you ate a plain white bagel. Peanut butter is also a source of protein, needed to build and repair muscles damaged during training.

How to add it to your diet: Get the natural kind with oil on the top and no added ingredients. Though high in fat, it's the good fat with no cholesterol. Peanut butter on whole grain or multi-grain bread makes a great breakfast.

9. Carrots

Why they're good for runners: Carrots are an excellent source of vitamin A, which helps promote a strong immune system. They fill you up but are low in calories, making them a great snack for runners who are watching their weight.

How to add it to your diet: Snack on baby carrots when you're hungry before dinner, so you can satisfy your hunger pangs and avoid overeating during dinner.

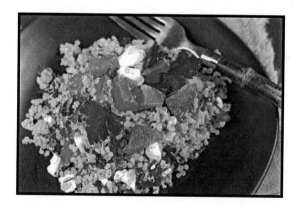

10. Quinoa

Why it's good for runners: For those runners who are bored with pasta, quinoa is a tasty alternative. Quinoa is not only packed with carbs, it's also very rich in protein. A six-ounce serving of quinoa contains 132 calories, 23 grams of carbohydrate, 4 grams of protein, and 2 grams of unsaturated fat.

How to add it to your diet: Cooking quinoa is very similar to boiling rice. It's an excellent side dish to have with fish or chicken. You can also eat it cold to go along with a salad.

By Christine Luff, www.running.about.com

Questions?

_____

_____

_____

_____

_____

_____

_____

Week 11 Workout Plan

Workout 1, 2 & 3

Brisk 5 Minute Warm-Up Walk

Jog 30 Minutes

5 Minute Cool Down Walk

Total Workout = 40 Minutes

Week 11 Conclusion

Remember that running is a great time to pray and talk with Jesus. It is also a great time to praise him, and that can be done through the music that you are listening to. Find some Godly music that you enjoy and load it on to your MP3, and delete anything that Jesus would not listen to.

Tip of the Week

Only one week to go— have you set your next goal? If not, set it now and be thinking ahead.

_____

_____

_____

_____

_____

_____

_____

_____

_____

_____

_____

Week 12: The Finish Line

Story

> "His Lord said unto him, 'Well done, *thou* good and faithful servant: thou hast been faithful over a few things, I will make thee ruler over many things: enter thou into the joy of thy Lord.'"
>
> — Matthew 25:21 (KJV)

I remember the first running goal I ever had. It was to run the Disney marathon in January 2007. My wife and I prepared for months to be able to cross that finish line. Date nights became running dates, sleep-ins became training runs, and nice hot showers became ice baths. We chose not to cut very many corners in our training. We were committed and focused on the goal at hand.

Race day came, and it was tough. The weather was hotter than normal (about 80 degrees in January) and I had the stomach bug. Seconds turned to minutes, minutes turned to hours, and hours turned into more hours. After more than five hours I felt like I just could not make it; my body had nothing else to give, and I was hurting badly.

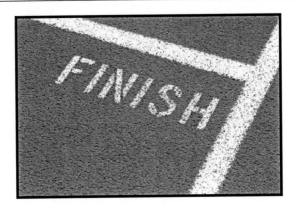

Anyone who has ever run a marathon will tell you that twenty miles feels as if you are only half way, and Disney's race directors knew this as well. You see, just as I was feeling like I had nothing else to offer, I began to hear music in the distance—not just any music—it was gospel music! Disney had lined the last half mile or so with a very large southern gospel choir. I do not remember what they were singing, but it was loud, and it was good. I went from feeling like I could not take another step to feeling like I was on top of the world and I could go another twenty-six miles. Crossing the finish line was unlike anything that I had ever experienced. I believe it is one of the few times that you can have tears of joy and pain at the same time.

I believe that this process paints a great picture of us as Christians. First, we have to make a commitment. For running that means signing up for a race, and for our Christian life the commitment is salvation. We have to be focused and committed. In both endurance sports and faith, this is hard—it is very hard. Sometimes it is painful, other times it's bliss. When we fall down, we must get back up, and when people say that you can't, you must say, "Yes, I can".

You see, for both of these processes, the finish line is the goal. Some of us may get there faster than others, but the important thing is that we get there. The feeling of finishing a race you have worked so hard for is like no other feeling, but it is only preview of the feeling we hope to have when we cross that final finish line and we hear the voice of our Father saying, "Well done, thy good and faithful servant."

By Mitchell Hollis

_____
_____
_____
_____
_____
_____
_____
_____
_____
_____
_____
_____

Discussion

In what ways has this journey, "Run for God," affected your life? _____

_____
_____
_____
_____
_____
_____
_____
_____
_____
_____
_____
_____
_____
_____
_____
_____
_____
_____
_____

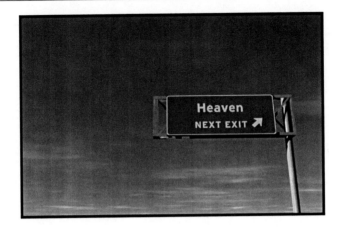

G et in the Word

Workout 1—Hebrews 12:1

_____

_____

_____

Workout 2—1 Corinthians 9:24

_____

_____

_____

Workout 3—2 Timothy 4:7

_____

_____

_____

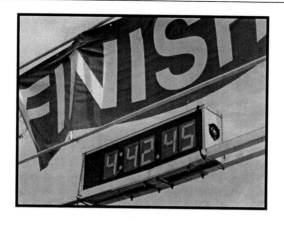

---

*R*ace Day

So, you've done your training for your first 5K or 10K—the race distances that are good for first-timers. As your race day approaches, you may have some questions and concerns about what to expect on race day. If you're fairly new to running, here are some tips for your first race day.

1. Pick up your race packet early

Pick up your bib, timing chip (if the race is using them) and goody bag the day before the race, if possible. This way, you won't have to worry about rushing to get it on the morning of the race. Also, you're more likely to get your desired race T-shirt size if you pick it up early.

2. Don't overdress

A good rule of thumb: Dress as if the weather is 15 degrees warmer than it is. That's how much you'll warm up once you start running. If it's cold, you can always wear warmer clothes while you're waiting for the race to start. Many races offer a gear check where you can store your bag of extra clothes for before and after the race.

3. Choose your pre-race food wisely.

Eat a meal at least one hour before the start of the race. Choose something high in carbohydrates and lower in fat, fiber, and protein. Stay away from rich, fatty, or high-fiber foods, as they may cause gastrointestinal distress.

4. Pin your bib properly.

Your race bib goes on the front of your shirt, not the back. You can use safety pins on all four corners of the bib to keep it in place.

5. Get there early

Arrive at the race site early to make sure you get a parking spot. Regardless of whether you're driving there or not, you'll also need time to pick up your number (if you haven't already), check your bag, take a warm-up jog, and use the bathroom (the lines may be long).

6. Line up properly

Don't line up near the front of the starting line. Faster, more seasoned runners don't like to weave around newbie (and likely slower) runners at the start of the race. Some races have corrals based on estimated pace or post pace signs. If not, ask runners nearby their anticipated pace. If it's faster than yours, move further back. It will be easier to fall into your pace if you're around people that run the same speed as you.

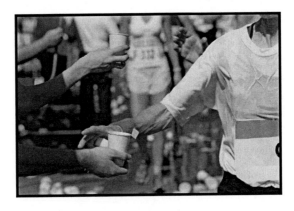

7. Use the water stops

Take advantage of the water stations on the course, and don't forget to thank the volunteers for handing out water!

8. Bring your support team

Invite your friends and family members to support you. Ask them to stand near the finish line so they can cheer you on at the end.

9. Aim to finish

Don't put pressure on yourself to achieve a really fast time for your first race. Finishing the race and enjoying the experience are excellent goals for a first-timer.

10. Don't wear the race T-shirt

Lastly, you'll most likely get a race T-shirt when you sign up for the race. Don't wear it until after you've completed the race. Not only are there superstitions associated with wearing it in the race, but it also makes you look like a rookie!

By Christine Luff, www.running.about.com

_____

_____

_____

_____

_____

_____

_____

_____

_____

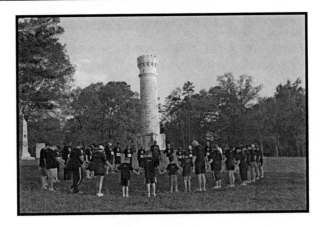

Questions?

_____

_____

_____

_____

_____

_____

_____

_____

_____

_____

*W*eek 12 Workout Plan

Workout 1

Brisk 5 Minute Warm-Up Walk

Jog 3 Miles

<u>5 Minute Cool Down Walk</u>

Total Workout = 3 Miles and 10 Minutes

Workout 2

Brisk 5 Minute Warm-Up Walk

Jog 2 Miles

<u>5 Minute Cool Down Walk</u>

Total Workout = 3 Miles and 10 Minutes

Workout 3

Walk for 20 Minutes

Race Day

Run 3.1 Miles

Have Fun

Praise God & Tell Others About Your Goofy Looking Shirt!

*B*reak it Down

Have fun and praise God for all that he has done for you!!

In Conclusion

I want to thank you from the bottom of my heart for taking this journey with me. It is my hope and prayer that not only did you gain a level of fitness you may not have had before starting this adventure, but that you gained a new level of spiritual confidence. I know that the Lord can do great things through you and I hope and pray that you will be sensitive to where the Lord may lead you.

Thank you again and God bless,

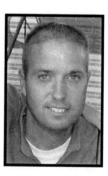

Mitchell Hollis, *Run For God!*

The Plan of Salvation

God loves you.

"For God so loved the world that He gave His only begotten Son, that whoever believes in Him should not perish but have everlasting Life."

—John 3:16

You are separated from God by sin.

"For all have sinned and fall short of the glory of God."

—Romans 3:23

Jesus died and rose again for you.

"But God demonstrates His own love toward us, in that while we were still sinners, Christ died for us."

—Romans 5:8

You can receive eternal life by accepting God's gift.

"That is you confess with your mouth the Lord Jesus and believe in your heart that God has raised him from the dead, you will be saved … For 'whoever calls on the name of the Lord shall be saved.'"

—Romans 10:9

"How can I receive Eternal Life?"

Admit

Your need for God's forgiveness and salvation.

Believe

That God can and will save you.

Call

On Jesus as your Savior and Lord.

Dear God, I know that you love me. I admit that I need forgiveness because I have sin in my life. I admit that I need salvation because I cannot save myself. I believe that you can and will save me if I ask. I believe that you died and rose again for me. I am calling on Jesus to be my Savior and the Lord of my life. I turn from my own way, and I turn to Jesus. Thank you for saving me.

In Jesus' name, Amen.

Bibliography

"Running the race before us," Douglas Bower, FCA Resources

"Running gear—The 'stuff' you need," www.therunnersguide.com

"Run your race," Jimmy Page, FCA Resources

Picture, www.tripleiron422.com

"How to choose running shoes," Linda Ellingsen, REI Outdoors

"Tip of the week," John Hanc, author of *The Essential Runner*

"Free to run," Jill Ewert, www.sharingthevictory.com, FCA Resources

"The hay is in the barn," Dan Britton

"Injuries / Injury Prevention," Christine Luff, www.running.about.com

"If you have to ask," Donna Douglas FCA Resources

"Basic Nutrition," Christine Luff, www.running.about.com

"Feed the Rabbit," Dan Britton

"Common Weight Loss Mistakes," Christine Luff, www.running.about.com

"Staying Motivated," www.therunnersguide.com

"The Right Race," Dan Britton

"Fat vs. Muscle," Ed Blonz, Ph.D.

"Road Race Etiquette Tips," Christine Luff, www.running.about.com

"The best food for runners," Christine Luff, www.running.about.com

"Race Day," Christine Luff, www.running.about.com

"Free to run photos" Asics America Corporation

"Various photos" Curtis Cox at clcphotography.com